A Handbook

David Baldwin
MB BS

Registrar in Psychiatry
St Mary's Hospital
London W2

Trainee General Practitioner
Hillingdon Hospital
Middlesex

Foreword by

Richard Smith
Assistant Editor
British Medical Journal

Blackwell Scientific Publications
OXFORD LONDON EDINBURGH
BOSTON PALO ALTO MELBOURNE

© 1987 by
Blackwell Scientific Publications
Editorial offices:
Osney Mead, Oxford OX2 0EL
(*Orders:* Tel. 0865 240201)
8 John Street, London WC1N 2ES
23 Ainslie Place, Edinburgh EH3 6AJ
52 Beacon Street, Boston
  Massachusetts 02108, USA
667 Lytton Avenue, Palo Alto
  California 94301, USA
107 Barry Street, Carlton
  Victoria 3053, Australia

All rights reserved. No part of this
publication may be reproduced, stored
in a retrieval system, or transmitted,
in any form or by any means,
electronic, mechanical, photocopying,
recording or otherwise
without the prior permission of
the copyright owner

First published 1987

Photoset by Enset (Photosetting),
Midsomer Norton, Bath, Avon
Printed and bound
in Great Britain by
Billing and Sons Ltd Worcester

DISTRIBUTORS

USA
  Year Book Medical Publishers
  35 East Wacker Drive
  Chicago, Illinois 60601
  (*Orders:* Tel. 312 726-9733)
Canada
  The C.V. Mosby Company
  5240 Finch Avenue East,
  Scarborough, Ontario
  (*Orders:* Tel. 416-298-1588)
Australia
  Blackwell Scientific Publications
  (Australia) Pty Ltd
  107 Barry Street
  Carlton, Victoria 3053
  (*Orders:* Tel. (03) 347 0300)

British Library
Cataloguing in Publication Data

Baldwin, David
  A handbook for housemen.
  1. Physicians—Great Britain
  2. Hospitals—Great Britain—
  Medical staff
  I. Title II. Hopcroft, Keith
  610.69'52   RA972

ISBN 0-632-01782-1

Contents

Acknowledgements, iv
Foreword, v
Preface, vii

Basics

1 First Days—Equipping Mind and Body, 3
2 Care of the Surgical Patient, 8
3 Care of the Medical Patient, 25

Topics of Interest

4 Cannulae, Intravenous Fluids and Transfusions, 41
5 Care of the Dying Patient, 47
6 Confusion, 50
7 Diagnosis and Management of Death, 53
8 Drug Charts, 57
9 Drug Reps, 61
10 Excuses and Ruses, 64
11 Insomnia, 71
12 Legalities, 75
13 Nursing Hierarchy, 80
14 Nutrition, 83
15 Peripheral Staff, 88
16 Practical Dilemmas and their Resolution, 91
17 Priorities, 99
18 Private Patients, 100
19 Referrals, 103
20 Relatives, 106

Contents

21 Routes of Exit, 110
22 Talking to Patients who take Overdoses, 115
23 Ward Rounds, 118

The Compleat Houseman

24 The Compleat Houseman, 125

Clerking

25 History and Examination Framework, 133
26 Abbreviations, 142

Index, 151

Acknowledgements

The authors wish to thank the following for their help in the preparation of this book: Professor Bowen, Sally Kay, Jonathan Miller, Denise Roberts, Jonathan Sackier, Richard Smith and all consultants, nursing staff and the single SHO who participated in the questionnaire.

Foreword

When I think back on my beginnings in hospital medicine, a lot of my memories are of terror. Lying awake in hideous bedrooms, waiting for the phone to go, and hoping that I would know what to do—or that some kind nurse would tell me. Getting up with the dawn at four in the morning, three hours before starting work, and practising surgical knots on a towel rail. And that terror I couldn't show to my superiors, nor even to my contemporaries—but only to my closest friends because I knew that they were just as scared. Maybe if I hadn't been able to share my fears and anxiety with them I would have gone the way of one contemporary who stabbed himself in the chest in a ward side room. Or perhaps I would have followed other young doctors who have just walked out of ward rounds and never been seen again.

But I must be wary of painting too bleak a picture because much of my housejobs I enjoyed enormously. My fondest memories are of companionship, often in the small hours, eating bacon sandwiches and watching a treated asthmatic finally fall into a grateful sleep. I remember, too, patients telling me wonderful stories—of fighting with the White Russians in Archangel, or of being rowed across the Firth of Forth in labour.

And if I'd been better prepared then I might well have been able much more quickly to quieten the anxieties and latch onto the pleasures. To a non-doctor it must seem extraordinary that you could spend six years at medical school (as I did) and yet begin your first job so inadequately prepared. 'What did the medical school teach you then?' they might ask, and I'd have to pause before answering. It taught me a mountain of facts, and it taught me how to dissect a corpse; it even taught me how to calculate creatinine clearance. But somehow it neglected to teach me the things that really mattered—like how to stitch up the forehead of a child, or what to say to a woman whose husband of 40 years had just died in her arms, or how to recognize, and admit, my own weaknesses and limitations. Indeed, my medical education even took some useful skills away from me. I knew how to say 'I don't know' before I went to medical school, but it took me 18 months of hospital work to learn it again.

When I did learn again it was one of my most useful lessons. I can still hear my friend (most of the really important lessons are learnt from people in the same boat rather than from superiors) saying: 'You know, you don't have to pretend that you know everything. You can always say, "I don't know what's causing your headache, but I'm pretty confident it's nothing serious. Come and see us again tomorrow if it's not any better."' Later from general practitioners I learnt to say to patients, 'I don't really know what's wrong with you. What do you think's wrong with you? Why did you come to see me?'

Maybe it's pie in the sky to think that the really important things could be taught at medical school. Perhaps just as you cannot lecture a 15 year old on adolescence and so let him skip 10 painful and, of course, pleasurable years, so you cannot teach many of the important aspects of being a doctor. They have to be learnt through experience.

But this book by David Baldwin and Keith Hopcroft will surely help the tyro. They point out, quite rightly, that much of the pain of those first days in a job can be alleviated by a close relationship with someone just ever so slightly more senior. A consultant is not much use, and nor is a registrar. But a sympathetic senior house officer is worth her weight in gold, and David and Keith have put that woman into book form.

Richard Smith
Assistant Editor,
British Medical Journal

Preface

Undergraduate medical education prepares students to be superb diagnosticians. To the houseman, working in the 'front-line', rather than the tactical manoeuvre department, this attribute is relatively redundant. The paradox which enables the new houseman to recite, for example, clinical features of myotonic dystrophy, the enzyme deficiencies in any number of obscure syndromes, and the multitudinous causes of peripheral neuropathy, whilst being hopelessly bewildered when faced with basic ward tasks such as correctly writing up fluid charts, preparing a patient for discharge, or dealing with death, renders him indignantly ignorant. Ironically, by the time the vast amount of theoretical knowledge acquired as a student is of real use, during senior house officer or registrar posts, much has been forgotten and requires re-learning and expanding via postgraduate examinations.

This chasm between the rather detached student training and the harsh reality of life on the wards became very apparent to us during our first days as junior doctors. With this realization arrived the idea for this book. We cannot claim that its contents are derived from years of experience or authority, since we have neither. However, we do have the recent memory of housejobs for which we were rather ill-prepared, some notions as to where a houseman's deficiencies usually lie, and the enthusiasm to distill these ideas into a guide designed to make housejobs more comfortable and rewarding for both houseman and patient alike. Thus, this book is best perused, at leisure, in the euphoric lull between passing Finals and commencing work on the wards.

For the sake of clarity, this guide is divided into distinct sections. The first deals with basic preparations for the post, and describes the junior doctor's role in the care of the medical and surgical patient. The second consists of a variety of individual topics of interest to the house officer, each dealt with concisely and included because we believe they are covered inadequately (over- or under-detailed, or even omitted entirely) in undergraduate education. We hope that the obvious drawbacks inherent in this part of the book—selection of the topics reflecting personal bias with, perhaps, a disjointed air due to the subjects being presented in alphabetical order—do not detract from the important information contained therein. Section three provides an insight into housejobs and housemen as viewed by nursing and consultant staff; the final part of the book covers medical symbols and abbreviations in common use, and provides a succinct reminder of the essentials of 'clerking': the basic skill of the house officer.

We are sensitive to the criticisms which a book of this sort might elicit. A comprehensive guide covering all eventualities is an impossibility, since no two housejobs or house officers are identical; our advice and opinions, then, must be interpreted with respect to the individual's particular post. Nonetheless, to provide some sort of basic framework for the fledgling doctor, we have occasionally assumed a rather dogmatic or simplistic stance where, in reality, 'hard and fast' rules may be difficult to apply. Written from the houseman's point of view it is perhaps inevitable that the guide appears at times to suggest a 'them and us' relationship between consultants and junior staff. Suffice to say that, without doubt, the vast majority of consultants are thoughtful, reasonable, and very supportive. In addition, we are fully aware that patients and medical staff may be female or male; our consistent use of the male gender in most cases should be regarded as economical prose rather than blatant sexism.

Finally, we would not be surprised if doctors who have successfully negotiated the hurdle of housejobs question the real need for a 'ward level' guide to housejobs. It is true to say that many of the 'tricks of the trade' are acquired rapidly by a mysterious, osmotic process, and house officers do appear most competent by the end of their pre-registration year. We would suggest that memories are short; the feelings of uncertainty, bewilderment and ignorance experienced by new housemen are almost universal and quite debilitating. If this book can dispel some of that fear, and increase the junior doctor's efficiency and standard of care, then the benefits reaped by housemen, nursing staff and patients should be ample justification for its existence.

Basics

I
*First Days—
Equipping Mind and Body*

Introduction

The present chapter is representative of our book in that it is of a very basic nature. It assumes that, frankly, you are entirely oblivious to the traumas of life as a houseman, and that you are therefore equally oblivious to mechanisms that might alleviate those traumas. Obviously, none of you can be so totally unprepared, but, for the purposes of this chapter, let us assume that you are—for herein may lie the odd hint or two that had not yet occurred to you.

It should be made quite clear that, almost without exception, young doctors experience some degree of misery during their first faltering steps in the profession. For many, housejobs are hectic torture. A minority, however, seem to adapt with uncanny ease. Such people may have one or more of the following characteristics:

1 An intimate familiarity with the particular post, e.g., via a previous attachment as a student or locum.

2 An intimate familiarity with the hospital and its mode of functioning (again, as a student or locum).

3 An awareness of the general role of a houseman through locum appointments at other hospitals.

4 A suitable degree of preparation for the post by accumulating information from various worthwhile sources.

5 Support in their role, especially from staff not too far elevated in the 'hospital ladder', e.g. Senior House Officers.

6 An extrovert and/or armour-plated personality.

7 Blissful ignorance.

It can be inferred from many of the above features that the disquiet associated with a 'first housejob' results from the newly-acquired doctor performing unfamiliar tasks in unfamiliar surroundings with unfamiliar people. This is normal. A partial remedy to this situation, alleviating the uncomfortable feelings of 'novelty' in those first few weeks, is preparation.

Preparation

It probably goes without saying that you should arrange to meet the doctor you are soon to replace. This meeting enables the 'experienced' houseman to impart essential information. (It should be noted that, often, a 'Ward Book' exists, listing information vital to the houseman's functioning, e.g. consultant's idiosyncrasies with regard to use of certain drugs, theatre-lists, etc. Even if this is available, however, such a gold-mine is rarely comprehensive.) In addition, you will have an opportunity to ask any questions or air any problems relating to the post which cause you particular concern. This 'fear-allaying' process is of great importance, especially to anxious, diligent types, and the sooner it commences the better. Quite apart from acting as a purely educational exercise, this meeting could enable you to be introduced to the relevant ward staff (or even patients) by your predecessor. Again, this plays a large part in removing the fear of the unknown when commencing a housejob. Such foresight tends to paint a favourable impression to all concerned.

At this stage, you ought to familiarize yourself with a timetable outlining your weekly routine so that you can envisage approximately how your work will be divided in time and place. Before you are left floundering alone on your first day, it is important that you understand the intricacies of the 'on-call' rota. Certain points regarding on-call duties should be clarified, such as the wards for which you are responsible and the accepted system of 'handing over' problem patients to the duty doctor.

In addition to this basic 'groundwork', as a fledgling houseman you should be reading a 'houseman's guide' of some sort (more specifically—this one) in preparation for your new job. This is best done on a sun-drenched beach somewhere; a good holiday is by far the best mind and body preparation of all.

First Days

Rules of day one

1 All administrative paperwork (contract-signing etc.) should, ideally, be completed before day one—if not, then as soon as possible, because you have quite enough to worry about on the wards.

2 Despite your inevitable nervousness, try to appear relaxed, pleasant and unhurried. This is impossible—however, the effort will be appreciated by those around you. First impressions are important, and never more so than on your first day on the ward. A good working relationship with the ward staff is essential if your job is to be at all enjoyable, and the foundation for this is laid at a very early stage.

3 At risk of appearing over-formal or eccentric, introduce yourself to the ward staff (especially Ward Sister) if you have not already done so. Unfortunately, in our experience, this has often met with bemusement or disinterest, but is worth a try.

4 Do not be afraid to appear mentally inert at times. Most nurses (especially senior staff):

(i) Know far more about the mechanics of ward-work than you.

(ii) In the realization that your mind is virginal in terms of ward 'know-how', will try to instil in you certain habits and attitudes. (Quite apart from contributing to your education, this tends to make the nurses' lives rather easier in the long run.)

(iii) Correctly despise arrogant know-alls intruding on what is predominantly their territory.

5 Establish the geography of the ward, and particularly the whereabouts of medical sundries (e.g. cannulae, syringes, stationery, etc.) as soon as possible, otherwise you will subsequently spend much time in frantic, often fruitless, searches. The exact location of the toilets is especially important on day one.

6 It is fine to appear an inane but amiable idiot to the nursing staff (at least initially) but it is a different matter when encountering your medical superiors. Again, ideally, you should have met these people prior to your first day. Try to exude intelligence and capability; their expectations will vary wildly but the fact that you at least *appear* fairly

mentally and physically 'together' will be of some relief to them (see below).

7 Look prepared and ready to work; clean white coat, stethoscope, notebook etc. Your mind is bound to be in disarray, so an organized body and accoutrements can only help. A word on notebooks and record-keeping might be in order here: *never trust your memory*—write everything down. Separate scraps of paper inevitably disappear amongst the white coat pocket jumble, so use a notebook. A mini clip-file (as championed by many a houseman) is ideal because, apart from being practical, it makes you feel like a proper doctor. Each page can be devoted to an individual patient, with, for example, relevant investigations and results noted down for easy reference, and the page removed and discarded when the patient is discharged, or dies. A prominent page of your notebook should be devoted to 'useful phone numbers', e.g. wards, secretaries, laboratories, etc.

Rules of subsequent days

1 Continue to be pleasant to all staff, no matter how difficult or even nauseating this might become. Results will soon be apparent, usually in terms of cups of coffee.

2 Attempt to visit as many departments of the hospital (pathology, X-ray, etc.) as soon as possible. In this way, the various cogs in the great machinery of the hospital will be able to put a face to your name. This pays dividends out of proportion to the effort required—investigations will be performed and results obtained that bit more rapidly, with a substantial reduction in the amount of arm-twisting necessary.

3 Never assume anything—the houseman is sometimes aptly known as the 'housedog', for it is he who is kicked should anything go wrong. The buck stops, inevitably, with the houseman (unless you are base enough to blame your medical student; see Chapter 10). Thus, it is in your best interests to be personally responsible for all aspects of your patients' care (especially with regard to investigations, results, drug treatment, etc.).

4 Anticipate—as you become more accustomed to your role, certain tricks of the trade will become apparent. These are usually specific to your particular post, but could include:

(i) 'Group and saving' surgical patients as soon as possible, e.g. when first seen in Casualty, even if operation is only a remote possibility (presuming, of course, that the proposed operation would probably require the availability of cross-matched blood). Similarly, procuring an ECG might be more convenient to you in Casualty rather than urgently, on the ward, just prior to the patient's transportation to theatre.

(ii) Filling out blood request forms in advance (e.g. the night before) if you are lucky enough to have the services of a phlebotomist.

(iii) Writing up discharge medication and dates for follow-up in outpatients as soon as you anticipate a patient's discharge—the nursing staff will adore you for this.

5 Keep patients' case and progress notes up to date. This is much appreciated by whoever eventually has the task of writing discharge summaries (it could be you!).

6 When in any doubt whatsoever about a certain problem, *ask* your immediate superior. He may well shout at you (particularly in the middle of the night) but he would shout rather more loudly if you were to make an ill-informed decision and thereby cause serious problems.

7 In general, keep a low profile. We are reliably informed that the housemen remembered most by consultants are those who have engineered some earth-stopping catastrophe. Thus, if your boss cannot recall your name, you are probably doing well.

With skill, judgement, foresight, luck, support, good physical and mental health, and more than 3 hours sleep per night, you should survive your housejobs. You might even enjoy them.

2
Care of the Surgical Patient

The majority of surgical patients are routine, or 'cold', admissions. Other modes of entry to the surgical wards include admissions from Casualty (i.e. emergency cases accepted by the 'on take' or 'receiving' team) or from out-patient clinics, and transfers from other wards or hospitals. The latter situations will be described later in this chapter. Although the care of the surgical patient is, in essence, the same regardless of route of admission, the following plan of patient management is tailored towards the patient admitted for elective surgery. Important variations occur in different surgical departments and, therefore, this is intended as a basic general guide.

Arrival of the patient

Invariably, the patient is greeted by the nursing staff when he arrives on the ward. Having been allocated a bed, he is then 'admitted' by a nurse; this is the nursing equivalent of the junior doctor's clerking. It enables information to be exchanged, such that the nursing staff elicit details necessary for the appropriate planned care of the patient, while the latter learns a little about the ward, the staff and the intended operation. In addition, the nurse takes a standard set of 'observations'—usually pulse, temperature and blood pressure, plus a dipstick urinalysis.

As the House Surgeon, you are the first member of the medical team to encounter the patient on the ward. It is worth remembering that, while the whole procedure of surgical management can become very routine to you, it may be a novel, bewildering experience for the patient. He may never have been in hospital before; he will probably not understand the roles of the various members of staff who he meets on the ward; he may have only a vague notion about what is likely to happen to him and will therefore probably be experiencing a good deal of anxiety. His initial impressions of you and your demeanour are vitally important. Naturally, an approachable, understanding and helpful doctor does a great deal to allay the patient's inevitable fears and ultimately fosters excellent doctor-patient co-operation. Hence, these positive attitudes should be apparent in your approach and communication from the outset. Before you even think about clerking the patient, you should introduce yourself (with a handshake), briefly delineate your own role in patient care, mention the names and status of the other members of the medical team (without being unnecessarily detailed) and explain your intended immediate action, which will probably involve clerking, venepuncture and the arrangement of other investigations. If you are the duty doctor covering routine admissions for another surgical team (e.g. at the weekend) then, to prevent subsequent confusion, you should mention to the patient that you will not be his 'permanent' doctor, but that the other surgical team will assume his care in due course.

Clerking the surgical patient

The surgical diagnosis specific to a patient who has been admitted for an elective procedure has usually been established some time earlier, often in the out-patient clinic. Bearing this in mind, the emphasis of 'routine' surgical clerking generally shifts from the requirement to establish a diagnosis to the need to ascertain fitness for operation. Concurrently, as you inevitably make some degree of enquiry into the history of the presenting complaint and, most certainly, examine the relevant part of the patient, the diagnosis is confirmed and the details recorded in the case-notes. It is a good idea to scan the patient's file prior to clerking, as much basic information may be gleaned in a short time; in addition, it is reassuring for the patient to find that you are already familiar with the fundamental aspects of his particular problem.

It is important, in some cases, to ascertain exactly what each individual has been told of his diagnosis prior to admission. Make some effort to obtain from your seniors a policy as to who gives the patient further details: it is mandatory that any information you give the patient is carefully recorded in the case-notes to prevent confusion for other practitioners.

The essential components of surgical clerking are the history, examination and special investigations. Points to be considered are as follows:

History

- Presenting surgical problem.
- Country of origin (significant because of possible haematological disorders).
- General fitness.
- Specific past or present medical problems in the light of impending anaesthetics and operations (e.g. cardiovascular or respiratory disorders, diabetes, bleeding tendencies, previous deep vein thromboses, etc.).
- Past and current medication, including the oral contraceptive pill.
- Allergies and intolerances (with particular reference to antibiotics and elastoplast).
- Previous operations (with special emphasis on any particular problems encountered, such as profuse post-operative vomiting).
- Smoking habits (patients should be informed, with rational explanation, that, regardless of their long term intentions, smoking is forbidden in the peri-operative period).
- Alcohol consumption (sudden cessation of a regular alcohol intake is a common cause of confusion in surgical patients, particularly elderly males). See Chapter 6.
- Social history, including occupation (of particular importance when discharge is contemplated).
- Family history of any relevant, or rare, medical conditions.
- Direct questioning—specific symptoms suggesting significant pathology, and which otherwise might have remained concealed, may be elicited by appropriate enquiry. Especially important are symptoms related to the cardiovascular or respiratory systems. Apparently trivial

complaints, such as a minor 'cold' might justifiably persuade an anaesthetist to postpone an elective operation.

Examination

- Presenting surgical problem (e.g. varicose veins, hernia, etc.).
- Apparent general fitness.
- Examination of body systems (although the nervous system is rarely examined in detail unless particularly appropriate) with special reference to the patient's heart and lungs.

A rapid check on history and examination taking and recording may be obtained by a glance through the 'Examination Framework', Chapter 25.

Investigations

The type and extent of standard pre-operative investigations vary according to numerous factors, including the patient's age, diagnosis, coincident medical problems and, particularly, ward protocol. Examples of the most commonly performed investigations in surgical patients are given below:

1 Haemoglobin—this value is nearly always required by the anaesthetist.

2 Sickle-cell test—this should be performed on all non-Caucasian patients.

3 Thalassaemia screen—this should be performed on all those of Mediterranean origin.

4 Urea and electrolytes—when indicated, for example in patients with renal disease or diabetes, on medication such as diuretics or digoxin, and those who may have a disturbance of electrolyte status because of diarrhoea or vomiting.

5 Liver function tests—if indicated, for example in those with a high alcohol intake (surgical admission in this case providing an opportunity for coincidental screening) and, often, before major abdominal surgery.

6 Cross-matching—a rough guide outlining recommended volumes of blood to be ordered for specific operations is given in Table 2.1. (NB your Consultant may well give you guidance in this area.)

Table 2.1. *Cross-matching*

Procedure	Units needed
Medium/major bowel surgery	2–4
Laparotomy	2
Cholecystectomy	2
Arterial cases	2–4
Aortic aneurysm repair	8
Amputation (except minor)	2–4
Prostatectomy	2
Major renal surgery	2
Mastectomy	2

Certain procedures involve only the possibility of transfusion requirement. In those cases, the patient should be 'Grouped and Saved' (see Chapter 4).

7 Chest X-ray—if indicated, e.g. heavy smoker, possible lung pathology, no previous or recent chest X-ray (NB Hospital policy plays an important role here).

8 ECG—usually required in patients over the age of fifty or in those with any history of cardiovascular disease.

9 'Special' investigations—described in detail later.

Obviously, such investigations should be arranged so that the results are available as and when required by the anaesthetist or your consultant. This may mean that, in practice, the venesection of your patient precedes thorough clerking, especially on wards where there is a very rapid turnover of patients, e.g. '5-day wards'. It may be possible for the patient to have certain necessary investigations performed immediately prior to admission. Thus, an elderly patient might be instructed to visit the X-ray and ECG departments on his way to the surgical wards. In this way, a chest X-ray and ECG can be obtained, when necessary, promptly and with a minimum of effort on your part.

Care of the Surgical Patient

Further pre-operative preparation

Routine surgical clerking provides the backbone of pre-operative preparation. However, many other important factors require careful consideration.

The anaesthetist in charge of a particular 'list' must be happy that each patient on that list is fit for a general anaesthetic. To this end, he (or his deputy) will usually review the pre-operative patients, with special regard to their cardiovascular and respiratory status. Despite this 'routine review', it is wise practice to draw an anaesthetist's attention to any pre-operative patient about whom you are particularly concerned. Thus, if further special investigations or preparations are subsequently thought necessary, they may be arranged in good time; similarly, if it is deemed necessary to cancel or postpone an operation, then this may be done at the earliest opportunity, causing as little inconvenience as possible to theatre, medical and nursing staff and, of course, the patient.

Most surgical patients will require premedication ('premed') prior to their operation. Often, the anaesthetist will be happy for you to write up a 'standard' premed in an uncomplicated case, usually dictated according to the surgeon's or anaesthetist's particular preference. Otherwise, the anaesthetist himself will take the responsibility for prescribing a suitable premed; the exact procedure varies from hospital to hospital. Examples of traditional premeds and their functions may be found in any anaesthetics textbook.

An area sometimes sadly neglected by the busy house surgeon is the imparting of an appropriate degree of information about the intended operation to the patient. The basis of this is the Consent Form, which must be signed by the patient prior to the procedure (see Chapter 12); it is stated on the form that the nature and effect of the operation should have been explained. This could, clearly, represent a minimal amount of information and it is essential for patient wellbeing that the houseman slowly and carefully details various aspects of the forthcoming operation. These should include:

1 As already mentioned, the nature and effect of the procedure (in

detail appropriate to the intelligence and interest of the individual patient).

2 Details of pre-operative care, including the investigations likely to be performed, the proposed time and date of the operation and the routine on the actual day of the procedure (e.g. the administration and effect of the premed).

3 Details of post-operative care, including the probability of the patient having a drip or blood transfusion (and the function of these incumbrences—many ill-informed patients will interpret the presence of a transfusion as evidence that something has gone horribly wrong), the likelihood of post-operative pain and therefore the requirement for analgesia, the duration of immobility and the likely time before recovery and discharge.

Emphasis on different areas of information will vary with individual patients, and some may require special advice or counselling (see 'Special Cases' later in this chapter).

In addition, it may be necessary to impart much of the above information to the patient's relatives.

As ever, during housejobs, anticipation of potential problems is essential. With regard to pre-operative preparation, a well-organized and diligent houseman will be fully aware, in advance, of impending operations (either by anticipating surgical management decisions concerning long term in-patients, or, in the case of other routine admissions, by perusing the ward diary, or similar, which usually gives information about forthcoming admissions). In this way, you will be aware, in good time, of any special preparation required in each individual patient. Similarly, you are able to anticipate post-operative complications specific to a particular procedure.

Forethought may also be applied to medication which is likely to be necessary post-operatively. If such drug therapy (e.g. powerful analgesics, usually scheduled for the first couple of post-operative days, followed by milder analgesics, and anti-emetics) is written up pre-operatively, then much time, trouble and discomfort may be saved when the patient returns from the theatre and you are busy in another part of the hospital. Some words of warning are necessary here, though: 'routine' prescribing can be dangerous, and therapy and dosage should be varied according to each individual's requirements. In addition, thoughtless administration of routine drug therapy may mask or distract attention from serious complications. For example, a patient may be treated *ad nauseam* with an anti-emetic for post-operative vomiting without anyone considering the possibility of a serious, remediable cause, such as intestinal obstruction. Therefore, although the need for certain medication can and should be anticipated, each case should be judged on its own merits and reviewed regularly.

At some stage during the planning of a set of operations, you (or your immediate superior) must prepare a 'theatre list', a programme delineating intended procedures to occur at a certain time and place. Ideally, this list is compiled when your other preparations are complete, but, in practice, the exact timing of its production is more a function of the deadlines of the particular departments to whom the list is delivered. These include the anaesthetic department, the operating theatre and the surgical wards. Like so much of the junior doctor's work, it is a case of discovering, or inheriting, a routine which is compatible with your workload and the demands of other individuals or departments.

The theatre list should contain the following information:

–Name of the surgeon due to perform the operations.

–Name of the theatre in which the operations are to take place.

–Appropriate date and time the list is expected to commence.

–Name, age, sex and ward of each patient.

–Intended procedure.

–Any special information, e.g. particular patient positioning, warning of Australia Antigen positive patients, the number of units of blood available, etc.

Your consultant may well have particular preferences in the 'running order' of his lists. It is prudent to become familiar with his idiosyncrasies at an early stage. However, a few 'hard and fast' rules apply. For example, procedures involving an infected area ('dirty' operations) are allocated to the end of the list, while operations on diabetic patients are usually placed early on the schedule. Many surgeons prefer to commence their work with a relatively minor procedure as a 'warm-up'; in addition, this gives the theatre staff time to prepare for the following, more complicated, operations.

Operative care

The operative care of the patient falls within the jurisdiction of the surgeon and the anaesthetist. Your role in theatre, if, indeed, your presence is required at all, ranges from onlooker or retractor-holder to performing minor surgical procedures under supervision.

At any point during an operation, you might be required to recall some aspect of the clinical history, examination or special investigations. It is, therefore, wise to commit all such information to the patient's case-notes rather than to trust them to memory.

Post-operative care

More often than not, you will be elsewhere when a patient returns to a particular ward after his operation. Immediate post-operative care is, therefore, the role of the nursing staff, and the exact form of this care reflects a combination of routine nursing process and special instructions from the anaesthetist or surgeon. You will only be involved in immediate post-operative management if there is some obvious urgent problem, such as haemorrhage or nursing observations veering alarmingly from the norm. Make it your routine to visit post-operative patients as soon as possible and to record your findings in the notes: this acts as an aide-memoire and assists other doctors who may be on emergency duty that night.

The post-operative care which impinges primarily on the house-surgeons workload involves the longer term management of the patient. Apart from 'post-operative complications', much of this work is quite routine. Basic points to remember are:

1 Fluid balance in patients with intravenous infusions (see Chapter 4). Ensure that the patient's fluids are written up well in advance and are appropriate to his requirements.

Care of the Surgical Patient

2 Post-operative investigations: in most medium or major-sized operations, there may be significant blood loss resulting in a decrease in the patient's haemoglobin level. A full blood count should, therefore, be taken on the first or second post-operative day, and measures instituted to organize an elective transfusion, should this prove necessary. Patients receiving intravenous infusions should have regular estimations of urea and electrolyte status.

3 Drugs: the patient's requirements regarding analgesics, anti-emetics, antibiotics and other medication should be reviewed regularly.

4 Communication: this process should, of course, continue, reinforcing the pre-operative preparation of the patient. Problems and anxieties should be identified and, if possible, allayed. It is also important to maintain a rapport with the patient's relatives, who may be confused or distressed by a person's post-operative physical or mental state. Communication between medical and nursing staff is vital: alterations in the day to day treatment plan of a post-operative patient must be relayed to the nurses if they are to be implemented effectively.

5 Other practical aspects: it is important to be aware of the intentions of your boss, as the nurses will turn to you for information should they be uncertain, for example, as to when stitches or drains should be removed.

The points outlined above deal with some fundamental areas of post-operative recovery. 'Post-operative complications' comprises a subject in its own right and is generally dealt with thoroughly in standard surgical textbooks. It is worth pointing out, however, that complications specific to certain procedures are most calmly and effectively dealt with when anticipated (as alluded to earlier in this section) rather than abruptly confronted. You should have a fairly standard plan in your mind for dealing with common problems such as post-operative pyrexia, confusion and pain. Careful review of the patient's subjective state and fluid and observation charts each day ensures that any complications are identified at an early, remediable stage.

Discharge

This subject is dealt with comprehensively in Chapter 21.

Special cases

Many patients will require investigation or preparation additional to the basic requirements which have been described in this chapter. As ever, consultant or ward policy dictates detailed management in these special cases, but examples, with general guidelines, are as follows:

1 Diabetics—the anaesthetist will probably expect a random or fasting blood glucose estimation to be included in the battery of pre-operative investigations. The aim of management is to maintain acceptable blood glucose levels during the peri-operative period when, obviously, the usual glucose intake and drug administration is interrupted. Generally, the anaesthetist will suggest how this aim is best achieved in each individual case. In many diet or diet+drug controlled diabetics, especially those undergoing a relatively 'quick' procedure, the only requirement is a slow-running dextrose infusion set up on the morning of the operation, with regular 'BM stix' monitoring of blood glucose. In other cases, a 'sliding insulin scale' may be used as soon as the patient is nil-by-mouth and has a dextrose drip *in situ*. For diet or diet+drug controlled diabetics, the insulin (a short-acting preparation) is administered subcutaneously according to four-hourly BM stix readings. Table 2.2 lists a commonly used regime:

Table 2.2. *BM stix readings and insulin dose in diet or diet+drug controlled diabetics*

BM stix	Dose of insulin (Units)
2– 7	0
8–10	5
11–13	10
14–22	15
> 23	20

In insulin dependent diabetics, a similar insulin is administered by an intravenous infusion pump according to hourly BM stix readings (Table 2.3).

Table 2.3. *BM stix readings and insulin dose rate in insulin dependent diabetics*

BM stix	Insulin dosage rate (Units/hour)
2– 4	0
5– 7	0.5
8–10	1.5
11–13	2.0
14–23	3.0
> 23	5.0

These regimes are continued until the patient is able to tolerate an adequate post-operative oral intake.

2 Chronic obstructive airways disease—patients with their respiratory system thus compromised will probably require extra pre-operative preparation, including:

- Lung function tests, such as FEV, FVC, FEV/FVC, PEFR.
- Arterial blood gas estimation.
- Pre- and post-operative physiotherapy.
- Sputum culture with antibiotic therapy if appropriate.

Such patients are prone to severe post-operative respiratory complications. These problems should be anticipated and treated vigorously.

3 Patients undergoing abdominal surgery—'antibiotic cover' and bowel preparation may be required, particularly with regard to procedures involving the large bowel. The antibiotic therapy is usually commenced with the premed and continued for 1 or 2 days after the operation (at the discretion of the surgeon). If a significant post-operative ileus is expected, then a nasogastric tube will be required. This is most conveniently inserted while the patient is under anaesthetic in theatre.

Patients in whom a colostomy or ileostomy is anticipated should receive ample pre- and post-operative counselling regarding the physical and psychological implications of a stoma. The help of a 'Stoma Nurse' is, in this situation, of great benefit.

4 Jaundiced patients—pre- and post-operative liver function tests are required. In addition, blood clotting tests should be performed pre-operatively. Many surgeons require the administration of intramuscular Vitamin K (even in the light of normal blood clotting results). Dehydration is an important danger and may result in the 'Hepato-renal Syndrome' (see standard texts). Thus, adequate hydration is essential and usually necessitates a pre-operative infusion and, sometimes, the administration of mannitol. Your superiors should provide guidance in these situations.

5 Patients undergoing cytoscopy—a pre-operative MSU must be obtained and infection, if present, treated appropriately. If the result of the MSU is not available before operation, then the patient should be 'covered' with a suitable broad-spectrum antibiotic.

6 Patients with particular cardiac lesions—patients with prosthetic heart valves, or a history of rheumatic heart disease, should sometimes receive antibiotic 'cover' during their operations, to guard against the possible development of bacterial endocarditis.

7 Patients with rheumatoid arthritis—the anaesthetist will usually require a cervical spine X-ray prior to the operation.

8 Certain 'at risk' patients—particular individuals (e.g. homosexuals, drug addicts) may need assessment of Australia Antigen, and possibly, HIV status.

9 Patients requiring 'marking'—in operations involving structures or areas represented bilaterally, the appropriate side must be marked, e.g. hernia repair, breast lump excision biopsy, etc. An arrow drawn onto the skin with a black marker pen is all that is required, and this is usually done on the morning of the operation, with instructions to the patient not to wash the mark away.

10 Patients requiring heparinization—by way of deep vein thrombosis prophylaxis, some units routinely administer to patients over the age of 50 years 5000 U of heparin subcutaneously with the premed, followed by 5000 U b.d. until mobility is restored. Women taking the oral contraceptive pill may be treated similarly when necessary.

11 Patients on medication—patients receiving certain forms of therapy, such as steroids or anticoagulants, present important and, often, rather difficult management problems. In these cases, the advice of the anaesthetist and/or other senior members of your medical team must be sought.

12 Operations involving other departments—certain procedures require the co-ordinated assistance of other departments of the hospital, such as the Pathology or Radiology departments. Examples include the need for a 'frozen section' histology examination during an operation, or per-operative ('on-table') cholangiography. You will need to develop a close liaison with the staff involved and a helpful, informative attitude if such procedures are to run smoothly. All requests should be made as early as possible, and, ideally, in person rather than by telephone: as ever, the small amount of effort required to appear diligent, efficient, friendly and interested, rather than representing yourself as a disembodied voice over the telephone, pays disproportionate dividends.

13 Patients likely to require intensive therapy post-operatively—patients who may be admitted to the intensive care unit (ICU) for an interim period (whether for hours or days) post-operatively should, ideally, be identified at an early stage in the pre-operative preparation. Such elective admissions to ICU usually comprise 'high risk' patients or those in whom a major procedure is contemplated. The value of this anticipation lies in the fact that an ICU bed may be reserved for the appropriate time-period (where possible). Lack of foresight in this situation, resulting in the unavailability of an ICU bed, can be dangerous for the patient, cause excessive work for the ward nursing staff, and is of extreme embarrassment to yourself.

The intensive care unit is a frightening and bewildering place to the uninitiated. A patient who is expected to spend some part of his post-operative recovery in such a department should have an idea of the sort of care in store for him. The most informative, and kindest, preparation involves a simple and leisurely guide around the unit so that he feels less threatened by the high technology and impersonal surroundings when he subsequently encounters them as the physically and mentally vulnerable post-operative patient.

Pre-operative check-list

Haemoglobin.
Sickle cell test/thalassaemia screen.
Urea and electrolytes.
Liver function tests.
Group and save or cross-match.
Other blood tests indicated, e.g. blood glucose or clotting screen.

Chest X-ray.
ECG.

Consent.
Information to patient and relatives.

Anaesthetic opinion.
Premedication and other appropriate medication on treatment chart.

Mark side.

Special
    diabetic or respiratory care
    antibiotic cover
    bowel preparation
    pre-operative hydration
    heparinization and drug problems
    additional X-rays e.g., cervical spine
    MSU
    Hepatitis B/HIV status in at risk individuals
    other departments, e.g., ICU, radiology, histology.

Theatre list.

Non-elective surgical admissions

As alluded to earlier, much of the management of the surgical patient is similar regardless of the route of admission to hospital. A few relevant points regarding 'non-elective' surgical admissions should, however, be mentioned.

The 'on-take' team is responsible for the management of emergency cases. Such patients are referred either by the casualty officer, after his initial assessment, or directly by General Practitioners in the community; in the latter situation, the GP usually telephones the registrar or SHO of the on-take team to request an urgent surgical opinion for one of his patients who is then transported to Casualty. Thus, the casualty officer is bypassed. It is essential to warn the casualty nursing staff of the imminent arrival of such a patient, and it is possible to order certain investigations (e.g. abdominal X-rays) in advance, when appropriate, with the request to be called when the patient is happily installed and the X-rays available. Further details may be found in Chapter 10.

Whether or not you are the first member of the surgical team to encounter the patient in the Accident and Emergency department will depend upon the immediate availability of your superiors and the urgency of the particular case.

In contrast to the elective admission, the 'on-take' patient will tax your diagnostic capabilities. You will probably be the person to initiate investigations and treatment, and much of this is best performed in the Casualty department (Sister and space permitting). Thus, blood samples may be taken, ECGs and X-rays performed, nasogastric tubes and intravenous lines inserted, and drug and fluid charts written up before the patient is taken to the ward. It is a wise policy to insist that all such admissions are kept 'nil-by-mouth' until seen by your superiors in case the decision to operate is made more rapidly than you had anticipated—unless, of course you are certain that an operation is not indicated. If you are feeling particularly baffled, technically incompetent, or fear that a situation is escalating into a life-threatening emergency, then do not hesitate to ask for help from the numerous medical staff who are inevitably present in the department, particularly if the other members of your surgical team are unavoidably delayed (e.g. in theatre or clinic).

Once the patient has been moved to the relative serenity of the ward, his 'work-up' can proceed at a more leisurely pace and your superiors informed of his admission. You will subsequently receive further instructions regarding the patient's investigation and treatment.

Occasionally, when your seniors are unavailable, you might be expected to 'arrange theatre' for an emergency case which will clearly require an urgent operation. This involves a series of telephone calls to inform theatre sister and the on-call anaesthetist of the particular patient and intended operation; the exact timing of the procedure (except in an absolute emergency, e.g. leaking aortic aneurysm) will depend upon the availability of theatre space, theatre staff, the on-call anaesthetist, and, also, the time elapsed since the patient last ate or drank, the latter being an important piece of information which you should elicit during your initial assessment in Casualty. In addition, the ward staff should be notified at an early stage so that a bed can be prepared in anticipation of the patient's arrival either directly from Casualty or via the operating theatre.

It often transpires that a patient admitted as an emergency, during your 'take' day, was recently under the care of one of the other surgical teams. In such cases, it is generally accepted that the admitting team provides any urgent treatment required and that subsequently, the patient is transferred back to the care of his original consultant.

Patients admitted from the outpatients clinic—a relatively rare occurrence—may have certain necessary basic investigations, such as blood tests, X-rays and ECGs performed on their way to the ward, thus effectively easing your workload.

Patients who are transferred from other wards or hospitals have, in most cases, already undergone thorough investigation. Therefore, assuming that inter- or intra-hospital communication is adequate, much of the essential information required for diagnosis and rational treatment will already be available; unnecessary replication of tests is costly, and unpleasant and tedious for the patient.

3
Care of the Medical Patient

Unlike their surgical counterparts, the majority of medical inpatients arrive as emergencies—though 'cold' admissions do occur, experience indicates that such individuals form only a comparatively small proportion of those occupying general medical beds.

Generalizing, there appear to be three 'types' of medical inpatient; those who arrive, de novo, as an emergency (e.g., a first episode of dyspnoea in an individual who subsequently becomes diagnosed as asthmatic); those who unfortunately suffer chronic, disabling disease subject to periods of remission, exacerbation, or complication (e.g., a patient admitted with a distressing 'flare-up' of rheumatoid arthritis); and those whose chronic disease has produced such profound physical, psychological and social disability as to require hospital admission.

These three 'groups' will be referred to as 'acute', 'acute-on-chronic', and 'chronic' patients respectively. Those patients admitted for 'social' reasons (often a great misnomer) will be included in the latter group, though will be discussed separately.

Obviously, the circumstances behind referral and subsequent admission govern the immediate management of the patient: you are unlikely to be thanked by the patient, his relatives, or senior members of your firm, if, when faced with an acute emergency, e.g., left ventricular failure, time is needlessly spent exploring the niceties of the patient's social circumstances. Similarly, a 'shock tactic' approach to individuals admitted for assessment and treatment of chronic disease is unlikely to be viewed sympathetically. What follows, therefore, should be considered only as a guide.

History

The reader is referred to 'History and Examination Framework',

Chapter 25. However, certain points require exploration in this chapter.

With 'acute' patients, the briefest history and examination that allows tentative diagnosis should be performed initially. The improvement in the patient's condition that hopefully follows urgent investigation and management will facilitate subsequent, more detailed, clerking. With 'acute-on-chronic' patients, more detailed assessment becomes necessary: evaluation of the frequency and severity of relapses should be performed; the therapeutic endeavours that have previously been successful, and those which have been unhelpful, recorded; elucidation as to how this attack might have been precipitated, and how it differs from its antecedents, explored; the patient's attitude to his disease and his carers noted. It is especially helpful to identify the extent of impairment by asking questions such as 'What could you do last week, that you can't today?'

In 'chronic' patients, a 'social' history is especially important: this should include evaluation of contact with friends and relatives; activities of daily living; difficulties encountered with present accommodation; extent of existing Social Services provisions, if any; finances and mobility. *Do not forget an alcohol history*.

Medical patients have frequently received a bewilderingly large number of investigations, diagnoses and treatments prior to your contact with them: as such it is often prudent to peruse the patient's notes before embarking on what might prove a confusing and epic clerking. Conversely, it is occasionally enlightening to approach the patients as if for the first time. Confusion may still occur after review of the patient's clinical records, for it is astonishing how sparse records of previous admissions may be, and how often discharge summaries are conspicuous by their absence. The latter frequently state 'see previous history', repetitively—searching may reveal no such initial information.

The 'systems review' section of your clerking should be as expansive as necessary: the brief outline of questions considered as mandatory for surgical patients is unlikely to be sufficiently informative for the assessment of factors other than fitness for anaesthesia. Exhaustive questioning is unlikely to be greeted by the patient, but it is surprising how frequently significant symptoms are not spontaneously proffered, these requiring 'winkling out' by direct questioning.

Examination

Regardless of the chosen speciality of the consultant responsible, it is negligent to regard his patients as possessing a particular 'system' (for example, central nervous system, gastrointestinal system, etc.), with secondary anatomical appendages, such as a head: all patients, medical and surgical, should be examined as thoroughly as is possible. Though amusement occasionally arises from such practice, for example when clerking a patient for avulsion of a great toe-nail, the medical defence societies would be hard pressed to defend omission of examination of the rest of the patient, should he die under anaesthesia.

One proviso exists, however: should the patient's physical condition be such that exhaustive examination would cause unnecessary distress, as might occur in an individual terminally ill due to disseminated carcinomatosis, it is obviously inhumane to subject him to extensive clerking, other than that necessary to relieve suffering.

Common sense governs the extent of *initial* examination, as stated previously; however, when the patient's condition has ameliorated as a result of therapeutic intervention, it behoves you that more detailed examination ensues. 'Medical' patients are more likely to be admitted as an emergency, and to display greater morbidity than their surgical counterparts, and as such more attention to detail, for example in the examination of the nervous and musculoskeletal systems, is required.

Examination of patients should be especially thorough when history-taking reveals inadequate information. Finally, it is expedient to scrutinize especially the 'system' favoured by your particular consultant: cursory examination of the cranial nerves is unlikely to be welcomed by a consultant neurologist.

Investigation

Pre-registration house officers commonly report feelings of frustration, irritation, and the sense of being overwhelmed, when faced with an accrued list of investigations to be performed on their consultant's patients. The rationale for many of these tests is frequently obscure, the nature esoteric, and the result equivocal; the perceived gain from subjecting a patient to investigations that are occasionally painful, dangerous and expensive, is often minimal. The following is not a luddite attempt to urge a return to a less technological age, but more an outline for the rational and appropriate use of investigation in patient care

Medical inpatients differ in fate from their surgical counterparts, the latter generally being subject to a limited number of tests that either indicate fitness for anaesthesia, or confirm clinical suspicion of a diagnosis in the 'surgical emergency'. It is interesting but somewhat sad that less attention appears to be paid to history and examination, and more to investigation, in the pre-anaesthetic 'work-up'. Medical inpatients are hopefully destined to avoid a trip to the operating theatre; their investigation should hence be less routine and more appropriate.

The 'ideal' investigation is easily performed, of minimal discomfort to the patient, reliable, valid, inexpensive, unequivocal, and should influence patient management: such a situation does not often exist. Though 'routine' full blood count, urea and electrolyte estimation, together with chest X-ray and ECG in patients aged over fifty years are advocated by many, consideration of the expenditure entailed is illuminating; money spent on one patient is money not spent on another, when faced with constraining regional and national health budgets. A balance has to be struck between negligence on the one hand, and overzealousness on the other; obviously, in this, as in all policy matters, the house officer's activity is governed by consultant attitude and preference.

One's position as a houseman is hence rendered somewhat difficult, when faced with angry laboratory staff enquiring as to why emergency evaluation of obscure parameters of clinical condition should be required, say, on a Sunday night. The answer to such pertinent questioning is *not* 'because my registrar wants it' but *either* 'recent studies indicate that . . .' *or* 'if you would like to discuss it with my superior

I suggest you contact him', and then stand back as the sparks fly. It is hard to appear convincing when defending requests in which one has little faith.

There is generally little kudos attached to the houseman's role in patient investigation, apart, that is, from your essential position as 'final common pathway' and repository of information, which should never be underestimated. The significance and practice of each pending investigation should be briefly delineated to the patient and relatives, should they be interested. It is sensible, however, to avoid prolonged discussion, which may not only reveal ignorance on your part, but also introduce an unnecessary level of anxiety to all concerned. Similarly, your role in the explanation of results is not to be undervalued—patients frequently prefer to be informed of the results by more senior members of the firm, but the person with whom they have the most contact, namely yourself, should be available to clarify and console when necessary. Beware of describing the results of investigations as 'normal'. Informing patients that blood tests, X-rays, etc. are normal can be terribly misleading, for gross pathology can exist in the presence of perfectly normal parameters.

The house officer is ascribed the role of provider of information, and is expected to pronounce and illuminate, oracle-like, on demand. Hence the great importance of accurate recording, and auditing, of the results of investigations in both the clinical notes and your pocket book. This obviously appeals to the more meticulous—a degree of obsessionality is a desirable quality in the houseman, and attempts should be made at its culture.

With the wealth of investigation that is now available, there is a tendency to lose sight of the basic purpose of investigation—namely, to influence patient management. Endless attempts to 'hunt' the primary carcinoma in elderly patients with disseminated secondaries who are terminally ill as a result, are inhumane and academic. The house officer can be of use in this matter, for though limited in medical knowledge, his greater involvement at a more personal level may allow him to persuade more senior members of the firm to adopt a more caring approach to patient management.

Management

It would be ridiculous to attempt an outline of the management of a cornucopia of diagnoses in the limited space that this book offers, indeed, such information should be indelibly printed on your consciousness as a result of Finals' revision. Your knowledge may have suffered the exponential decline so characteristic of post-Finals euphoria, and it is prudent to carry, at all times, a medical emergencies handbook, thus enabling you to appear capable, with only minimal delay, at times of need. Less acute management problems can be resolved after consultation of standard textbooks if necessary.

What follows is an outline of the management of a limited number of broad situations, each frequently occurring during your time as a house officer.

'Crash calls'

Recent studies have drawn attention to the poor knowledge and performance of house officers in the management of cardiopulmonary resuscitation, CPR. This observation, though regrettable, is hardly surprising, since most medical students' experience of CPR is limited, and house officer preparatory courses at medical school tend to be inadequate or nonexistent.

Similarly, it is not surprising that carrying the 'crash' bleep is an anxiety-provoking situation: one's first few days in this invidious position are likely to be characterized by a constant fear that the bleep may actually go off—presumably ignorance and inexperience each have roles in increasing one's level of autonomic arousal. Repeated physical presence at crash calls gradually causes a reduction of anxiety: what follows attempts to allay such fears, through acquaintance with *basic* techniques of CPR, prior to the need to actually perform it.

Care of the Medical Patient

Procedure of cardiopulmonary resuscitation

1 Establish the diagnosis, by noting the absence of carotid and femoral pulsation associated with collapse and unconsciousness: it is ridiculous to auscultate the heart in the general brouhaha and panic engendered by the crash call.

2 If possible, ensure that the patient *is* 'for cardiopulmonary resuscitation'.

3 Ensure that the patient is on a firm surface, with as much surrounding space cleared as possible.

4 Establish that the airway is clear—the patient will invariably have vomited so use a sucker as soon as it is available. Remove false teeth and other debris.

5 Simultaneously, commence external cardiac massage and adequate ventilation either by mouth or Ambu bag (using 100% oxygen if possible). Cardiac massage should be performed at approximately 60 compressions/minute: it is no longer considered necessary to maintain synchronous massage and ventilation—more importantly, ensure that both procedures are performed adequately. This should render the patient less blue, and should produce a palpable pulse.

6 Immediate management complete, now ascertain that the anaesthetist has been called, and that the 'crash trolley' has arrived by the patient's bedside.

7 Note the time.

8 Patients may be maintained in this state of suspended animation for up to 20 minutes: hence time is now available for more considered decisions. Points 1–7 should have been reflex response. Ensure intravenous access: it is uncommon to find a complete absence of peripheral veins—if this regrettable situation has arisen, a central line will be necessary.

9 Run in approximately 100 ml of bicarbonate as soon as a drip is functioning—thereafter be more circumspect, it is a common failing to be overzealous with the bicarbonate bag.

10 An anaesthetist should now be installed at the head of the bed, if not, you should insert an endotracheal tube. Failure to intubate should

not precipitate repeated attempts—better to continue to use the Ambu bag.

11 Check that the endotracheal (ET) tube is *in situ* by blowing down the tube and listening to the chest. This obviously requires a period of silence from attendant individuals.

12 Fasten the ET tube to the patient's face as gently as possible, then attach the tube to a 100% oxygen supply.

13 Deliver a DC shock with the defibrillator as soon as it arrives—any delay is life-threatening if the patient's cardiac activity is ventricular fibrillation: if asystole, no harm will be done. The conventional defibrillators contain oscilloscopes to provide a visual analogue of the patient's cardiac rhythm.

The stage is now set for the on-call medical senior house officer or registrar to assume control and decide which inotropic, chronotropic, and antidysrhythmic agents to use. Central lines, intracardiac injections, pacing and thoracotomies may be contemplated—your role is to ensure that the practicalities of resuscitation are being maintained.

Certain aspects of the procedure outlined above require elaboration. Obviously, it is important to clearly record in the nursing and medical notes when a patient has been considered as unlikely to benefit from cardiopulmonary resuscitation. Practically, it is expedient to familiarize yourself with defibrillators *prior* to your first day as a houseman: you may be required to use it in your first hour! Certain defibrillators do not possess an oscilloscope, and in these cases, obviously, ECG leads should be attached to the patient as soon as possible in the event of cardiopulmonary arrest. When using a defibrillator to deliver DC shocks, anyone touching the patient or bed is likely to be the recipient of an electrical surprise they would be better without. On a similarly practical note, you will find that the insertion of an endotracheal tube is not an easy procedure: it is therefore necessary, though somewhat macabre, to practise intubation after unsuccessful attempts at resuscitation.

Finally, remember that crash calls are physically and mentally exhausting, not only to the staff involved, but also to the patient, should he recover. They also constitute a stressful event to all other

Care of the Medical Patient

patients, and their relatives, should they be present on the ward. Do not underestimate the impact of your, often very audible, activities on ward consciousness.

'Not for emergency resuscitation'

Patients die in hospital, usually in one of three ways. Certain terminal events occur surrounded by frenetic activity from a flurry of white coats. Other patients die, or are allowed to die, as a result of terminal illness, peacefully in their sleep. Many, however are 'actively managed' to an extent that falls short, usually arbitrarily so, of cardiopulmonary resuscitation.

The rigeurs and necessities of resuscitation are described in the preceding section: the involvement of house officers in the management of those patients allowed to die with the minimum of intervention is described in Chapters 5 and 7.

It is enlightening, somewhat surprising, and occasionally perturbing, during one's first few days as a houseman, to be besieged by senior members of the nursing staff, requesting that certain patients be designated as 'not for resuscitation'. Patients so described were, on occasion, identified by the inclusion of a red circular sticker on the clip of nursing observations at the end of the bed. Thankfully, such public display of intent (or lack of it) is now avoided—red dots being transferred to the 'Kardex' in some cases.

The decision to designate a patient as unsuitable for resuscitation should preferably never be made by house officers, it being more prudent for senior staff to commit themselves after discussion with all concerned parties. It is hard to imagine staff, relatives or patients wishing to prolong distress and suffering in those condemned to irreversible terminal illness, as may be the case in disseminated carcinomatosis, endstage chronic obstructive airways disease, and motor neurone disease. It is important to take *all* opinions into account; not least the patient's, who may often express a desire not to be resuscitated that would be churlish and inhuman to ignore.

Having made the decision not to resuscitate the patient, it is obviously mandatory that clear instructions are written in the medical and nursing records. Dreadful chaos will otherwise ensue.

Greater difficulty arises in those patients who are considered as suitable for 'active' management, to a specified limit. For example, the management of a moribund dehydrated, pyrexial 93 year old with bronchopneumonia initially appears straightforward. Consider, however, the following dilemmas, for where does active management stop? Is simple reduction of temperature and rehydration sufficient? If so, should the latter be achieved by nasogastric or intravenous means? Should antibiotic therapy be instituted? If so, by oral or intravenous route? Finally, what if the patient recovers from a presumed toxic confusional state to reveal that he is suffering from irreversible Alzheimer's disease?

There are, of course, no didactic answers to the above questions. Consideration of each patient, on individual merits, is the rule. The patient's age alone should only very rarely be used to govern intended extent of management. It is prudent to speculate on the possible effects that one's actions determine, *prior* to their institution, in the same way that consideration of the necessity of investigations is required prior to their implementation.

Social admissions

It is sad that insufficient community resources exist to prevent the unplanned admission of patients in whom no medical cause for admission is found. Examples of such patients include those admitted due to illness in relatives normally responsible for their care, and elderly patients admitted when their electricity supply has been cut off. It is sadder, however, that many such 'social' admissions are characterized by derogatory assessment and care from medical and nursing staff. Such patients are frequently destined to receive less attention, and more likely to develop morbidity as a consequence of hospital admission, than those perceived by the carers as having greater medical need. This situation, therefore, is not without paradox for though resentful of 'social' admissions, frequently, minimal effort is made by the responsible medical team to ensure continuity of care when the patient is re-established in the community, and consequently increased morbidity necessitates re-admission.

Remember that the distress associated with admission is generally greater in 'social' admissions than in those patients occupying hospital beds as a result of more acute illness, in whom loss of self-esteem is usually, though not invariably, absent. Reassurance is probably the most important aspect of management in social admissions.

Until such time as the socioeconomic climate changes, it seems likely that 'social' admissions will account for approximately one-fifth of inpatient beds. Management of social admissions is often astonishingly simple—and rewarding—for provision of additional social input is often all that is required, for example, weekly visits by a district nurse, or attendance at old people's luncheon clubs. It should not be the fate of these individuals to wait for long-term residential care, forgotten at the end of the ward, developing life-threatening chest infections and painful pressure ulceration. Resources for the rehabilitation of the elderly and infirm are always likely to be more restricted than those for widely-publicized high-technology units.

It makes sense, therefore, for an accurate and detailed history to be taken, and for repeated examination to occur in patients admitted for 'social' reasons. Liaison with the social work and occupational therapy departments should occur at an early stage. Geriatricians have great experience in dealing with unlimited demand on limited resources; their expertise should not be ignored. A 'Resource Book', listing available social service and voluntary organization provisions, should be kept up-to-date and consulted regularly. The relevant general practitioner should be informed of the patient's progress, and is occasionally able to oblige in rehabilitation by admitting to 'cottage' hospitals.

Experience indicates that discharge from hospital is often delayed for reasons that are initially obscure, for example the discharge of an elderly lady with only minor venous ulceration, in whom daily visits from a district nurse had been organized, was delayed inordinately whilst waiting for the patient's gas supply to be reconnected: a phone call to the responsible engineer resulted in same-day reconnection. It pays to be 'on-the-ball' in the rehabilitation of these patients, whose management should always be 'active'.

'Problem-orientated' approach to the care of long-term patients

Medical inpatients are frequently victim to multisystem pathology, the associated morbidity necessitating complicated and prolonged management. It is not surprising therefore that the reasons for admission, initial diagnosis, and results of investigations become 'lost' in the detailed mess of medical notes. Fashioning order out of chaos is a prerequisite for competent management.

Many consultants advocate the following system, in an attempt to clarify the continuing care of their patients (Table 53.1).

Table 3.1. *Example of system employed to clarify patient care*

Subjective	Breathlessness on exertion
Objective	Dyspnoeic at rest Moist inspiratory crepitations at base of both lung fields
Assessment	?Incipient left ventricular failure
Plan	Chest X-ray ECG Institution of diuretic therapy Investigation of cause
Education	Necessity of medication Recognition of symptoms as requiring medical intervention

The presence of multisystem pathology renders the example in Table 3.1 somewhat simplistic, but each category may be usefully outlined under major headings such as:
1 Left ventricular failure

Care of the Medical Patient

2 Maturity-onset diabetes
3 Hypertension
4 Depressive illness

Such an approach should not replace time-honoured methods of clerking on admission, but constitutes a useful addition to continued care of long-term patients.

Topics of Interest

4
Cannulae, Intravenous Fluids and Transfusions

A drip renders someone a patient in the same way that a stethoscope or white coat signifies a doctor. Such symbolism is commonly reinforced by the media, and the patient encumbered with an intravenous infusion is, inevitably, in the eyes of his relatives and friends, 'really ill'. This mystical aura surrounding these patients seems somehow to rub off on the more junior medical staff, at least initially. While the theory of fluid balance and its associated problems are taught to medical students, 'ward-level' intravenous infusions, their use and abuse, are all too rarely mentioned.

Cannulae

Undoubtedly, the most common problem encountered with intravenous cannulae is their efficient and painless insertion into a suitable vein. Possible methods of alleviating this torture, for both doctors and patients, are detailed in Chapter 16. However, a few additional points deserve mention:

You are rarely in a position to demonstrate thoughtfulness and compassion when approaching a patient with a long, sharp needle which you are about to stick into him. The insertion of an intravenous cannula provides one such opportunity. Having gently explained the procedure, you ask the patient whether he is right- or left-handed. With a sympathetic smile, you then attempt to insert the needle into a vein on the non-dominant arm, explaining, as you do so, that you wish the patient's dominant hand to be left unhindered by drip-lines. This is usually appreciated by the patient, so much so that he might even remain unaware of the pain you are inflicting. Shaving the arm (see Chapter 16) shows similar forethought.

It should be noted that, if the veins on the dominant side appear considerably 'easier' than on the other arm, then the above advice should be totally disregarded. Many doctors feel that the instillation of a small amount of local anaesthetic around the appropriate vein is justified prior to this procedure. If any blood tests are coincidentally required, then a suitable sample may be obtained via the intravenous cannula prior to its connection to the drip set. This saves the patient further discomfort.

Intravenous cannulae, once successfully inserted, reach the end of their useful life when they fall out, are pulled out, 'tissue' (i.e. the fluid they transmit enters the tissue around the vein) or cause local inflammation (phlebitis). The latter two conditions are best treated by local application of ice, elevation, and oral analgesics or anti-inflammatory agents as appropriate. Some 'tissued' intravenous fluids (e.g. cytotoxic drugs) can cause horrendous problems, such as skin necrosis; if in doubt, consult. Drip failure due to inadequate securing of the cannula to the skin, resulting in the cannula simply falling out, is depressing and unnecessary. Therefore, assume responsibility for securing your own cannulae—especially in a confused or restless patient, or one with few suitable veins.

The mechanics of 'running a drip through', i.e. the preparation of the infusion 'giving set', is usually the domain of an obliging nurse. Nonetheless, it is worth familiarizing yourself with the anatomy of the infusion apparatus as you will undoubtedly one day find yourself expected to cope with it yourself.

Intravenous fluids

As already mentioned, fluid balance forms a well-recognized part of the undergraduate curriculum. Excessively detailed and theoretical instruction leaves the new doctor totally bewildered when he discovers that he has ten fluid-charts to write-up in his first half-hour as a surgical houseman. Simplicity is the key. Gross misconceptions will soon be noticed and rectified by your superiors.

The most obvious example of a patient requiring an intravenous infusion occurs in the post-operative period of a medium or major abdominal operation. After such a procedure, the inevitable paralytic ileus renders the patient unable to obtain his fluid requirements orally. In this situation, the 'standard' regime comprises 3 litres of fluid per day, usually in the form of:
2 litres 5% dextrose
1 litre isotonic (0.9% or normal) saline
Each litre is administered over a period of 8 hours

In addition, 60 mEq of potassium are needed over each 24-hour period *after* the first post-operative day (there is internal release of potassium on the first day or so after an operation). This is usually provided as 20 mEq with each of the doses described above: bags of 5% dextrose or normal saline with 20 mEq of potassium are manufactured for this purpose.

Such a scheme should maintain the patient on a biochemically stable course during the post-operative recovery. The regime is recorded on the fluid balance chart usually found at the end of the patient's bed. The following points should be borne in mind:

1 Fluid regimes for most other situations may be easily calculated from this most basic of schemes

2 Adequate fluid input should be confirmed clinically by monitoring the patient's hydration and urinary output.

3 Care should be taken not to cause fluid overload, especially in the elderly (many authorities suggest that the elderly should usually only receive 2 litres of fluid per 24-hours, although other factors, such as weight and general constitution, should be considered).

4 Adjustment should be made to the scheme described above according to supplementary fluid input or output. For example, a post-operative patient who is beginning to tolerate oral fluids should have the volume administered orally, approximately subtracted from his 'standard' intravenous requirement. Similarly, those losing extra fluid (e.g. via drains, or sweating because of fever) will require appropriate supplementary fluids.

5 It is generally recommended, though rather uncommonly im-

plemented, that patients receiving intravenous fluids should have their serum urea and electrolyte status checked every other day (or more frequently if necessary).

6 Intravenous maintenance over a period of weeks rather than days is a totally different situation, whereby adequate nutrition must be administered in appropriate fluid form. In the commoner, short-term therapy, maintenance of fluids and electrolytes is all that is required. The long-term administration of intravenous infusion, in the absence of any oral intake, comprises 'total parenteral nutrition', (see Chapter 14).

7 Occasionally, an infusion will be maintained merely to provide access to a vein (e.g. for intravenous drugs). In this case, the minimum amount of fluid should be prescribed to keep the drip functioning. In practice, this usually amounts to approximately 1 litre every 12 hours. A more satisfactory method, which does not necessitate the administration of unnecessary volumes of fluid, and provides greater mobility for the patient, is to insert a cannula in the usual way, then maintain it in a functioning state by twice daily 'flushes' of 500 units of heparin.

8 Fluid balance (and, sometimes, the insertion of cannulae) in children is a subject in its own right. Rational intravenous therapy cannot be extrapolated from the recommendations described above. If a child requires an intravenous infusion (e.g. after an appendicectomy) then it is essential that you seek the advice of your superior, or a paediatrician. When you have experienced such a situation on a few occasions, you should feel confident enough to manage the problem yourself, although it is always wise to err on the side of caution and consult if in any doubt.

Transfusions

Blood transfusion is merely a special case of intravenous fluid therapy. 'Whole blood' transfusion is most commonly encountered in the operating theatre or in an emergency (e.g. acute haemorrhage) although, in the latter case, initial treatment comprises plasma expanders until cross-matched blood is available. Thus, it is relatively unusual for the houseman to be involved with 'whole blood' therapy; generally, he is simply required to ensure that the appropriate volume is ordered and available for elective or emergency operations.

The more common situation involves the patient who is anaemic and who requires 'routine' blood transfusion to elevate his haemoglobin concentration to acceptable levels. Such is the case, for example, in the otherwise uncomplicated patient whose post-operative full blood count reveals a low haemoglobin caused by blood-loss during operation. Rational treatment consists of the administration of 'packed red cells' (i.e. plasma-reduced blood, produced so as to provide the maximum amount of haemoglobin without overloading the patient with unnecessary fluid volume). As a general (and often inaccurate) rule, 1 unit of packed cells will elevate a patient's haemoglobin concentration by approximately 1 g/dl. Some important practical aspects are discussed below.

1 While in the process of taking a venous sample for a full blood count in a patient who may be anaemic (or who may conceivably require blood transfusion for any other reason, e.g. during operation, in the near future), it saves you time, and the patient injections, if you also withdraw enough blood for 'group and saving'. Should that particular patient subsequently require a transfusion, a simple telephone call to the laboratory is all that is required to arrange the appropriate volume of blood at the most convenient time.

2 As it is impractical to remain on the ward until the blood actually arrives, most housemen set up the infusion in advance, using, for example, a 500 ml bag of normal saline to keep the intravenous line functioning (written on the fluid chart as 'TKVO', 'to keep vein open', or as a 6-hourly infusion, to be removed and replaced by the blood when the latter is available). Dextrose should not be used for this purpose because the subsequent mixing of blood and dextrose in the giving set can cause clotting and result in blockage of the apparatus.

3 In an 'elective' transfusion, the packed cells are usually administered as slowly as possible; the standard infusion time is 4 hours/unit. A

slower rate may result in a clogged giving set while a more rapid regime may result in fluid overload, particularly in the elderly. Because of the latter problem, many doctors routinely prescribe 20 mg of frusemide orally, to be given at the beginning of each unit, so that excess fluid is rapidly removed from the circulation via the kidneys.

4 The nursing staff perform frequent observations of pulse and temperature on a patient receiving a blood transfusion. Thus, these procedures are best instituted as early in the morning as possible; a nurse will not thank you for enforcing her to wake a patient regularly throughout the night and nor will the patient.

5 'Transfusion reactions', usually in the form of pyrexia or mild urticaria, are common and serious problems arise only rarely. A ritual search for the cause of the pyrexia is inevitably instituted; if you are satisfied that nothing particularly untoward is going on, then the standard treatment for such reactions (e.g. slowing the drip rate and administering an anti-pyretic or anti-histamine) may be commenced. Obviously, in the event of a serious transfusion reaction, then the infusion should be stopped immediately, appropriate therapy started and your superior contacted.

5
Care of the Dying Patient

Care of the dying patient is generally ignored in undergraduate teaching. Though reference may be made, in pharmacology lectures, to the need for regular prescription of opiate analgesics in the relief of intractable pain in terminal illness, an holistic approach is rarely taught. Presumably, it is felt that this approach evolves through clinical experience, as indeed it does, but initially you will be ill-prepared, and uncertain what to say, and what to do, in the care of a dying patient. It is quite conceivable that you might confront such a situation on your first day as a houseman—obviously, clinical experience will then be at a minimum, so the following guidelines should be of assistance.

The basic aim of the nursing and medical staff must be to ensure that the patient is kept free from pain, and able to live a fulfilling and dignified existence, satisfying his remaining wishes. Patients may complain of a number of physical problems, such as pain, nausea, vomiting, breathlessness and incontinence; these must be treated effectively, with the minimum of investigation, to enable the patient to live his last days in comfort. In addition, it is almost certain that you will detect anxiety, and depressive feelings amongst the terminally ill. Understandably, most patients have a fear of death, at least initially, however, much of their trepidation may be related to fears of placing an intolerable burden on those around them, or to pain, or loss of dignity. Depression is common, and may be considered a normal grief reaction; such depressive feelings are commonly displaced onto the care-givers, with subsequent bitterness and hostility towards relatives, nurses, and doctors—you will find this disturbing, but later come to realize its origin, and act accordingly.

Thus, the first stage in the management of dying patients is the relief of distressing physical symptoms. Of equal importance, is the establishment of a rapport in which the patient may discuss his illness and feelings as much as he wants, or is capable.

Much is said in the debate as to whether patients should be told of their illness, its complications and duration; in our experience, it is best to let the patient lead the way in discussions of diagnosis and prognosis. Withhold information until the patient indicates that he is prepared to know, then gradually tell him; reticence on your part would then only encourage feelings of distrust. You will constantly be surprised, and relieved, that when (after endless deliberation on your part) you eventually decide to start indicating the prognosis to a patient, he will declare 'I know I am dying'; frank, but concerned discussion can then occur, with great relief to all. Understandably, the cardinal rule in terminal care is that every case is different; judge each patient's needs individually, dogmatic rules or techniques inevitably result in the loss of a sympathetic, personal approach.

It is worth remembering, however, that certain wards, specifically radiotherapy or oncology wards, have fairly defined policies as regards telling the patient the truth; these will need to be observed as much as is appropriate.

It is of paramount importance to keep relatives' views in sight: no one will thank you (except, on occasion, the patient) should you decide to weigh in and break a conspiracy of silence. However, much of relatives' well-intentioned desires to withhold information from the patient stems from ignorance of the severity, complications, and treatment of the patient's illness, hence, informed discussion with all concerned parties is the key to honesty in the management of the terminally ill. Relatives' fragile conspiracies in withholding information from the patient often prove difficult to maintain; unfortunately, such fragility may be revealed by those least involved in the care of the terminally ill, for example an innocent and unintentional remark from a ward domestic might instill great suspicion and fear in the mind of the patient.

Often, after adequate treatment of physical complaints, it is possible to transfer the patient to the caring environment of the family home, or failing that, a hospice, if the patient indicates a preference to leave hospital. Re-admission to the ward should be guaranteed, if

Care of the Dying Patient

this is considered necessary by the patient or his care-givers. Hospitals, it must be stated, are generally not a nice place in which to die.

Various stages occur in the acceptance, by the patient, of his imminent death; these are classically referred to as 'denial', 'anger', 'bargaining', 'depression', and, finally, 'acceptance'. Obviously, these are only terms for the wealth of feeling and emotion that occurs in everyone, and any stage may be especially prominent, or contemporaneous with others. Simple conversation will reveal the stage in the patient's perception of his illness. It is tempting, as a new houseman, to avoid such conversation: this attitude probably arises from uncertainty as to what is required, difficulty in choosing the correct word and appropriate expression of concern, together with feelings of inadequacy, for medical education teaches us to preserve life, rather than ease death. By simply imagining a reversal of roles, with yourself in the hospital bed, you should begin to realize what is required in probably the most difficult, but potentially most rewarding part of your job.

6
Confusion

The descriptive term 'confusion' is so commonly used as to be rendered meaningless. This is not surprising since the state of confusion, i.e. an inability to think clearly, is part of normal experience for many—including patients and housemen. A partial impairment of consciousness (with features such as disorientation, disturbance of memory, hallucinations and delusions) is better described as an 'acute confusional state', thus distinguishing clinical condition from popular experience. 'Patient confused' is a common and inadequate description of a regrettably frequent phenomenon—acute confusional states occurring in approximately 10% of patients in general medical and surgical wards during their admission.

For this reason, nurses will frequently call you to assess patients found in compromising states of undress, and exhibiting bizarre behaviour, who on examination are found to be grossly disorientated and deluded.

The first step in the management of such patients is concise and accurate assessment of the mental state. Impairment of consciousness, manifested by, for example, poor attention and loss of short term memory is usually obvious, and frequently worse at night: disorientation is invariable. Additionally, many other features can be found: behaviour may range from overactive, aggressive and irritable, to retarded and mute; repetitive mannerisms occur frequently; thoughts may be slow and muddled, delusions prominent; abnormal visual perceptions, including misinterpretations of the surroundings, and hallucinations, may be present.

Subsequently, an attempt is made to elucidate any physical causes. There is not sufficient space for exhaustive classification, but disorientation occurring immediately post-operatively is usually a result of the combined effects of analgesia, anaesthesia and hypoxia. Delayed dis-

Confusion

orientation has many causes, notably various forms of failure, whether it be cardiac, respiratory, renal, or hepatic in origin. Infection, including septicaemia, is a commonly implicated factor, especially in the elderly. Intracranial causes, for example, meningitis, head injury and raised intracranial pressure are rare but life-threatening. Iatrogenic factors are common and administration of drugs such as anticholinergics, analgesics, digoxin and benzodiazepines, or, alternatively, withdrawal of drugs including alcohol and paradoxically, benzodiazepines, are common causes of disorientation. Hypothermia and hypoglycaemia should be considered, especially in 'at risk' groups, such as elderly or diabetic patients.

It is apparent, therefore, that when faced with a 'confused' patient, simple physical examination, including elementary measures such as ascertaining the patient's temperature, listening to the chest, and feeling for a full bladder (another common cause), together with casting an eye on fluid balance and drug charts, may well allow a causative factor to be elucidated, and appropriate management instituted. Unfortunately, the clinical picture is frequently far removed from this idyllic representation—exhaustive investigation commonly fails to reveal any abnormality and a sense of despair would occur, were it not that acute confusional states show a tendency to ameliorate suddenly, leaving the houseman perplexed as to what exactly had occurred.

Problems in diagnosis include distinguishing between organic and functional causes of acute confusional states; it is worth remembering that illusions, visual hallucinations, and profound disorientation are virtually pathognomic of organic disorder, and that a depressed mood is a common early manifestation of organic brain syndromes. Features such as ataxia, dysarthria and incontinence are uncommon manifestations of functional psychosis.

Obviously, treatment of any underlying cause will be the cornerstone of management—but symptomatic relief is required to alleviate the distress that disorientated patients cause to themselves, relatives, fellow patients, and nursing and medical staff. Such measures include the reduction of anxiety: you should attempt to explain to the patient what is occurring (assuming that you know) even though he may appear oblivious to reassurance: nursing by familiar staff in a quiet room is ideal as are visits from hopefully reassuring figures such as close relatives. It is prudent to restrict drug prescription, and certainly avoid polypharmacy—nevertheless, daytime relief of distress, without causing drowsiness, and night-time induction of sleep, may be required.

Confusion in yourself is unlikely to be that occurring in an organic brain syndrome, more probably being the result of the inability to think clearly, mentioned earlier. Such a state is produced by the volume of work foisted upon you, and its associated stress, a new environment, the acquisition of a disconcertingly large number of colleagues manifesting the same degree of disorientation, and your generally virgin state in hospital matters. Simple supportive measures, for example the maintanence of a notebook with timetable, telephone numbers, patients' results, etc., is essential and is described in Chapter 1.

7
Diagnosis and Management of Death

Most recently qualified doctors have little experience of dead people other than those preserved in the all-pervading aura of formalin within the dissecting room. The recently dead patient presents a fairly simple and common problem.

Diagnosis

Let us assume that you are bleeped in the middle of the night (which is when these events seem to occur most often) to be informed that a patient has just died. (This obviously refers to the anticipated death as opposed to an unexpected demise—in the latter case, if the patient is discovered rapidly enough, then a 'crash call' is more likely.) Very occasionally, the Nursing Officer on duty might be prepared to pronounce the patient dead, in which case you continue to slumber having been notified of the event. However, you must remember to both identify the body in the mortuary and complete the relevant forms in the morning.

However, in general you are forced to leave your bed to confirm, medically, that the patient is actually deceased. This might sound somewhat absurd, but can sometimes be a source of concern (patients have been known to take one breath every 30 seconds—admittedly, this tends to precede death but can be rather unnerving). It is worth pointing out that this crude diagnosis of death which follows should not be confused with the much more complex diagnosis of 'brain stem death' which belongs in the realms of medical ethics and intensive care medicine. Death is confirmed by:

1 Fixed and dilated pupils
2 Absent carotid pulse
3 No breath sounds over 1 minute

4 No heart sounds over 1 minute

Note: to this list, some doctors add: no response to painful stimuli (e.g. pressing your thumb forcefully over the patient's sternum); retinal changes (interruptions in the blood columns in the patient's retinal vessels as viewed via the ophthalmoscope).

Very rarely do doctors actually listen to the breath and heart sounds for 1 complete minute. Sixty seconds can seem an awfully long time when listening to a manifestly dead patient's inert heart and lungs. However, it is not good practice to cut corners in this situation.

Management

Having confirmed death, it is your duty to record it:
1 In the patient's case notes, usually written as:
Date/time—called to see
   —pupils fixed and dilated
   —°carotid pulse
   —°BS ⎫
         ⎬ over 1 min
   —°HS ⎭
Patient pronounced (or certified) dead

Some housemen become rather blasé about this procedure to the extent that a patient's death is recorded as follows:

Day/time—called to see
   —patient dead
   —RIP

This is not to be recommended.

2 In the ward death certification book (not to be confused with issuing a death certificate). Your signature may be required (although the procedure varies from hospital to hospital) usually carbon copied onto three detachable slips of paper; one remains on the ward, one is affixed to the patient's notes and the other accompanies the patient to the mortuary.

Management of Death

The next step is to inform the relatives. If the death has been expected for some time, then they might already be in attendance. More commonly, they are contacted by telephone, usually by the nursing staff, unless you express a specific desire to be the person who breaks the bad news (which might be appropriate, for example, if you had previously had long, supportive discussions and established a good rapport with specific relatives).

At this stage, it is worth considering whether or not anyone else ought to be informed of the death—the consultant handling the case if the death was unexpected, or, perhaps, if it was a private patient. Generally, however, it is sufficient to inform the appropriate 'team' of the death the next morning. It is also prudent to notify the deceased patient's GP.

Completion of the death certificate is usually carried out the following day; this task is usually quite simple, but, if there is any doubt about the correct manner of completion, then your immediate superior or administrative Patients' Affairs Officer should be contacted.

Essentially, you may complete the death certificate if:
- you were the doctor in attendance during the deceased's last illness
- you know the cause of death
- you are happy that the Coroner need not be involved

Instances in which the Coroner *should* be involved are:

–where the cause of death is not clear

–where the doctor has not attended in the last illness or within 14 days of death

–in criminal abortion

–accidents or injuries of any date contributing to death

–alcoholism (acute or chronic)

–following anaesthesia or from operative procedures before recovering from anaesthesia or following injury

–drug addiction, overdose or mishap

–ill treatment, i.e. starvation or neglect

–industrial disease

–obscure infant deaths

–from causes for which the deceased has received pensions or disability awards

—deaths of persons in legal custody
—if there is any suggestion that relatives are dissatisfied with treatment
—poisoning
—septicaemia following injury
—stillbirths from 24 weeks maturity
—violent or unnatural deaths not covered by the above list.

In such cases, the death should be reported to the Coroner as soon as possible. Commonly, the Patients' Affairs Officer will do this for you by giving the appropriate details to the Coroner's Officer (a police officer attached to the Coroner's Court). If the Coroner decides that a post-mortem is necessary, then the certification procedure will no longer be your responsibility.

Sometimes, your superior might request a post-mortem after the death of a particular patient. Written consent from a relative, next-of-kin or executor is essential; forms for this purpose are available in most hospitals. In addition, provided you are satisfied with the clinical cause of death, the death certificate should be completed there and then if possible.

If, in a 'non-Coroner's case', the patient's relatives decide to dispose of the body by cremation, then you will be required to complete 'Form B', the certificate of medical attendance, of the cremation form. This includes 18 questions about the care, mode of dying and cause of death of the patient and may only be completed if you have seen the body after death. New housemen often find the receipt of a fee for this minor service rather distasteful. However, most doctors find that they can quickly overcome this moral hurdle and soon regard cremation money (or 'ash cash' as it is popularly known) as one of the few perks of the job. It is important to note that the cremation fee is taxable. Thus, you should keep a record of this income, especially in view of the fact that the Inland Revenue has only recently realized that junior doctors are regularly in receipt of such fees.

8
Drug Charts

Medication to be administered to a particular patient is recorded in the individual's 'drug chart'. Thus, these charts provide both a means of ordering treatment and a record of the therapy given to an 'in-patient' during his stay in hospital. Their exact format varies but they all have certain essential components. The usual subdivisions of a drug chart are as follows:

1 'Regular medication'—here, therapy to be administered on a regular basis is tabulated. This generally comprises the drugs the patient was taking on admission (unless some are withdrawn as a therapeutic manoeuvre), with any additions deemed necessary by the receiving medical or surgical team.

2 'As required medication'—any treatment likely to be required intermittently is prescribed in this section. Examples include analgesics and night sedation, although some prescription sheets have a separate space for the latter.

3 'Once only medication'—this comprises presumed one-dose treatment, such as a single injection of intravenous frusemide in a patient with left ventricular failure, or a dose of a powerful analgesic in a patient with severe pain which is likely to be of short duration.

Pre-medication drugs may be recorded here or in a specific pre-med section of the chart.

4 'Variable dosage medication'—this section is used to record drug requirements which might vary from day to day in terms of the precise dose appropriate for the patient, e.g. warfarin or prednisolone.

5 'Allergies and idiosyncracies'—these are generally recorded on the cover of the chart.

6 'Discharge drugs'—here, drugs which the patient is to take home are ordered.

7 'Intravenous fluids'—in a few cases, intravenous fluid requirements

may be recorded on the drug chart. More commonly, however, these regimes are written on the 'Fluid Charts'.

8 'Special diets'—some charts provide space for recording the necessity for a special diet, e.g. diabetic patients or patients taking monoamine oxidase inhibitors.

There is a very ill-defined boundary between therapy which must be specifically prescribed on the patient's chart and treatment which may be administered via a verbal message to the nursing staff. For example, many hospitals require that orders for glycerine suppositories or certain enemas should be recorded on the drug chart before such treatment may be administered. Similarly, oxygen, at the desired percentage, necessitates specific prescription.

The structure of a drug chart allows the actual administration of each dose of a particular drug to be recorded (in the form of the nurse's initials). For any drug, the following points must be specified:

- generic name of the drug
- dose
- formulation (when appropriate)
- starting date (and date for treatment to be stopped, if necessary)
- frequency of administration
- route
- special instructions (e.g. 'with food')

Each order should be signed by the prescribing doctor.

Drug charts are often a minefield of medical abbreviations and jargon (see Chapter 26). A few specific examples of common prescription formats follow:

Regular: nifedipine SR 20 mg bd, O, duration$|_\infty$ (= nifedipine slow release, 20 mg twice a day orally, indefinitely).

As required: paracetamol T̄–T̄T̄ 4 hly PRN, O, to max. 8/day (= paracetamol one to two tablets four hourly as required orally to a maximum of 8 per day).

Once only: 15/1/85, 7.30 pm, frusemide 40 mg, IV (= frusemide, 40 mg, given intravenously at 7.30 pm, 15/1/85. Such 'single shots' are sometimes known as 'Stat. doses').

On the ward, drug charts are kept filed together in a single folder, or, rather more usefully, with the other charts on a clipboard at the end of the patient's bed, where they are easily accessible during ward rounds.

The accurate and efficient writing up of medication on the drug chart is a habit you will acquire quite painlessly in your first few weeks as a houseman. It should become a reflex action to compile such a chart for each new patient after the initial clerking. Certain prescriptions become 'automatic':

- A mild, as required, painkiller, such as paracetamol. This is, essentially, a prophylactic, the prevention in this case orientated towards eradicating the need for nursing staff to call you to prescribe a painkiller should the patient suffer, for example, a slight headache.
- Night sedation, e.g. temazepam 10 mg nocte PRN. For a more detailed consideration, see Chapter 11.
- In post-operative patients—anti-emetics to alleviate the vomiting caused by the general anaesthetic.
- Other specific cases, e.g. glyceryl trinitrate for the patient with known ischaemic heart disease, heparin 'flush' for the patient with an intravenous cannula *in situ*, etc.

However, in all such routine prescribing, the warnings outlined in Chapter 2 should be noted.

Regardless of your pharmacological prowess, it is wise to become familiar with the dose, actions and side-effects of a limited number of drugs for use in the appropriate clinical situation. This personal formulary will reflect your own idiosyncracies and those of the hospital pharmacy. An up-to-date British National Formulary should always be available on the wards for reference, especially with regard to correct dosages and possible drug interactions.

Whenever prescribing medication, always consider carefully the particular patient in question. For example, a patient with dysphagia might tolerate more readily an analgesic in syrup rather than tablet or capsule form; a cachectic patient requiring parenteral antibiotics will suffer unnecessary pain if repeated intramuscular injections (often of quite large volume) are administered, and will, in the long run, appreciate the painless access offered by an indwelling intravenous cannula. Various ploys may be used to overcome route of administration problems in 'nil-by-mouth' patients, in whom certain analgesics may be given sublingually, antibiotics in suppository form per rectum, and so on. Particular care should always be taken when prescribing for the elderly, the young or the pregnant, or for those patients with hepatic or renal impairment.

It is a wise policy to set aside time once or twice a week to simply check through the drug charts of all your patients. This regular review will ensure that medications are given in the appropriate dosage and formulation for the correct time, and prevents the 'forgotten' patient from being subjected to unnecessary drug therapy. In addition, all drug charts are perused regularly by a 'ward pharmacist'. Apart from quietly and politely pointing out any mistakes you might make, this person can provide helpful suggestions and advice when you are faced with a pharmacological conundrum.

Discharge drugs are best ordered on the patient's prescription chart as soon as you have a proposed date for his discharge from hospital so that the correct medication may be obtained in good time from the pharmacy. In practice, this entails writing the 'TTAs' on the chart during, or immediately after, a ward round.

A knowledge of the anatomy of drug charts and the correct manner of prescribing medication is essential. Common sense, diligence and accuracy in this area delight the nursing staff, who, otherwise, are obliged to call you to the ward for trivial and irritating prescription errors or omissions. It must be said, though, that drug charts are not very interesting.

9
Drug Reps

Finals over, and having gained provisional registration with the General Medical Council, it is your probable fate to receive a veritable cornucopia of communication from pharmaceutical companies. Product has to be marketed.

Pharmaceutical companies exist primarily to discover, research, manufacture and market drugs. Many drugs, initially perceived as universal panaceae, are rejected during this process, such that approximately only one-thousandth of synthesized molecules eventually reach the stage of clinical evaluation. A company marketing one new drug every couple of years is considered successful. Brief glances at the prices of their shares rarely reveal, however, impecuniosity amongst pharmaceutical companies. This is undoubtedly because their product is undeniably useful—it is also due to effective merchandising.

Such marketing occurs through a multiplicity of media channels: for example, communication in person, video, film and written word. Information is presented in a palatable fashion; garnished with selectively supporting evidence; and finished off with an impressive array of free gifts, viewed by the naïve as useful aide-memoires, by the cynical as an exercise in bribery and corruption.

The relative seniority of the target market governs the strategy and tactics adopted by the company. Consultants may receive informed discussion of the relative merits of a number of drugs, useful in their chosen sub-speciality, with supporting evidence from carefully conducted controlled clinical trials. Gifts that may be proffered, though not necessarily accepted, may include medical, or other, equipment. Housemen are considered to possess only a very small voice in the hubbub of policy decision in wards and hospitals, and are not usually regarded as a particular prime target for drug reps, attempting to persuade a 'firm' to adopt a new product. They are instead viewed as having their own needs: the product must be presented as easy to administer, and effective: gifts to housemen, therefore, are also essentially practical—for example pens, pads and diaries, all emblazoned with the product name.

Representatives of pharmaceutical companies show considerable variation—most are university postgraduates in natural sciences; some, however, are medically qualified; such individuals generally being directed towards the more senior echelons of the medical profession. Reps are usually allocated to a particular region of the country, or alternatively to marketing product for a particular area of the medical world: most receive defined salaries, with additional remuneration, on a commission basis—it is in their interests, therefore, to be forceful, seductive, and persuasive.

Your interests are different, but should not preclude mutually-satisfying compromise. Reams of useful information may come your way, increasing your knowledge, and consequently improving the service that you are able to offer your patients. The interview itself offers opportunities, that may not previously have existed, to demand supporting evidence for the claimed benefits of the drug on sale, and to exercise greater objectivity in the assessment of drugs, than was possible in the blinkered vision of undergraduate days. Many of the free gifts are useful, and, providing they do not unfairly influence your decision to use a particular drug, may be accepted. Interest, enthusiasm, and informed discussion on your part is likely to guarantee your successors similar benefits—providing, that is, the pharmaceutical company feels its product sales to be adequate.

The most hallowed forum in the interactive process is the Drug Lunch. The food on offer is probably more palatable than that available in the hospital canteen. The Drug Reps on these occasions appear to have given up attempts to make themselves heard over the munching that ensues. The following snippet of *genuine* drug lunch chatter illustrates the points nicely:

Drug Rep: '. . . so I'll think you'll agree . . .'
Doctor A: 'Wow! This cheese is terrific!'
Drug Rep: '. . . that drug X represents a significant advance . . .'

Doctor B: (mouth full): '. . . Mmmm, yeah . . . What is it?'
Drug Rep: 'Essentially an angiotensin con- . . .'
Doctor A: 'Brie I think'
Drug Rep: '. . . -verting enzyme inhibitor'
Doctor B: 'Oh, right. Hey, where did you get this cheese?'

To avoid these situations, resort to film and video, should facilities be available, commonly occurs. Unfortunately, the darkness that is required makes eating difficult. The demonstration is initially impartial, later becoming more partisan: discussion follows; an awkward silence precedes an undignified rush for the free gifts.

It is hard to understand how such a clichéd format could have survived so long—perhaps, simply because everyone needs to eat. Certainly, other forms of persuasion appear to be increasingly fashionable. Realizing that the prescribing habits of junior doctors are largely governed by consultant preference, pharmaceutical companies now frequently offer *services,* without specific product marketing: money may be donated to the doctors' mess; a stethoscope overhaul service instituted; medical and ward equipment provided; non-promotional educational videos shown. The doctors remember the *company* name, not that of its product.

Seeing Drug Reps should never be considered a nuisance: if feeling tired, or excessively busy, inform them as such and suggest another time when you anticipate a greater degree of freedom. After all, it is in everyone's interest . . .

Except, perhaps, the patient's. It is probably incorrect to view pharmaceutical companies' attempted control of doctors' prescribing habits as remnants of the animosity that occurred during the separation into distinct guilds of apothecaries and physicians in feudal times. It is unfortunately true, however, that the companies exercise great selectivity, in presenting information, to support their product. This is understandable: product has to be marketed. Remember not to be deceived—you should have your patients' interests at heart.

10
Excuses and Ruses

Inevitably, once the mass of information contained within this book had been sifted and categorized into appropriate sections to produce something approaching an ordered guide for otherwise uninformed new housemen, there remained a few topics of interest which did not fit comfortably into the existing chapters. These have been thrown together here under the guise of Excuses and Ruses, a collection of advice and manoeuvres, some well-tried and tested, others of rather dubious merit, but all potentially useful.

Nothing emphasizes the gulf in responsibility and workload between houseman and clinical student more than each party's attitude towards the humble paging device, or 'bleep'. To the medical student, whose activities are only infrequently interrupted by its chirping, the bleep is something of a status symbol. In contrast, it soon becomes the proverbial bane of the houseman's life, bleeping without any regard to time or circumstance, and is justifiably viewed as harbinger of that exquisite torture, sleep deprivation. Little can be done to decrease the frequency with which you are paged, apart from improving your overall efficiency with ward work and, perhaps, educating the nursing staff. The shrillness of each individual bleep may, however, be adjusted, the judicious application of adhesive tape across an appropriate area of the device rendering its calls rather less shocking. Some bleeps may actually be turned off by the user, but this practice is, for obvious reasons, absolutely condemned.

You may, with time, find a few positive uses for your own bleep. For example, it is quite simple to arrange for the nursing staff to page you at a pre-determined time, thus legitimizing your premature exit from some situation which you would otherwise have had to endure; meetings with drug representatives or the occasional obnoxious relative, and some 'lunchtime seminars' might fall into this category. Modern, deluxe paging systems possess a visual 'display', rather like that of a calculator, which indicates the telephone number of the caller when you are paged, thus bypassing the time-consuming system mediated directly via the switchboard. Many enterprising individuals have taken advantage of this high-technology by devising various codes designed to facilitate communication. Thus, a bank of zeros across the visual display could indicate, for example, that the curry has arrived. Similarly, when wishing to contact your registrar quite urgently, you might prefix your dialling number with some simple code (such as '00'), which had been agreed upon beforehand. In this way, your registrar will realize that you require his advice and will, in theory, answer his bleep quite promptly.

It has been known for junior doctors to misplace their bleeps. This usually occurs after a series of arduous nights on duty, when the exhausted houseman clambers gratefully into bed, throwing clothes, bleep and white coat onto the floor where they coalesce with the heap of dirty laundry, books, magazines and half-eaten canteen snacks which tend to accumulate in these circumstances. Typically, in the morning, the bleep is nowhere to be found. It may be easily located, in rather circular fashion, by the doctor bleeping himself and 'homing in' on the concealed device.

A nocturnal 'bleep' heralding some emergency on the ward, may allow situations where the sacred history/examination/investigation protocol might usefully be inverted. In the delay between your bleep interrupting your sleep and your bleary-eyed arrival on the ward, the nursing staff could be performing ECGs, contacting a radiologist or preparing infusion sets—if asked politely. Occasionally, it may transpire that such action was unnecessary or inappropriate once you are 'on the spot' and able to assess the situation via a formal history and examination. Generally, though, the institution of important diagnostic or therapeutic procedures by the nursing staff, at your request, prior to your arrival is ultimately of benefit to both doctor and patient.

On 'take' days, when you are the junior doctor responsible for emergency admissions, tend to invite various ploys aimed at reducing the inevitably massive workload. Most of these manoeuvres are ill-judged or ineffective. It is a common fallacy amongst new housemen to believe that a full ward, at the beginning of a 'take' day, implies an inability to accept urgent admissions; some juniors, under this misconception, make no efforts to precipitate a patient's discharge when it might, in fact, be appropriate. In reality, as the houseman soon discovers to his dismay, a lack of beds on his wards simply results in him having to seek room for his emergency admissions on other wards. Obtaining beds in this way is a highly time-consuming administrative task, and caring for 'outliers' (as such patients are known) adds disproportionately to the day's labours as it incurs extra time journeying to and from wards and involves caring for patients in unfamiliar surroundings with nursing staff of a different medical or surgical speciality. Therefore, it is imperative to establish the number of vacant beds on your wards during the early morning round on 'take' days, and, where possible, to engineer their availability.

Another common mistake involving emergency admissions is to enter prolonged debates over the telephone with GPs who request an urgent senior opinion. All too often, housemen are guilty of interrogating the GP, demanding information which is either irrelevant or could be obtained at leisure later, when the patient is seen in the Casualty department. These tactics serve only to make the houseman appear both ignorant and inexperienced. If a GP has taken the trouble to visit a patient and then contact the appropriate team at his local hospital, rather than simply send the patient, unheralded, to Casualty, then he is at least entitled to a senior medical or surgical opinion. Your role should merely be to record the patient's name, age, address, sex and, if possible, hospital number, the name of the GP and the tentative diagnosis; it is reasonable to request that a letter detailing medication and other relevant past medical history should accompany the patient. You should inform the Casualty Department of the patient's imminent arrival and request any action or investigations (such as the retrieval of old case-notes, urine testing, chest X-ray or

ECG) which might usefully be performed before you arrive to assess the patient yourself. In addition, it is courteous to warn your superiors of the expected admission.

Dealing with emergency cases in Casualty is a rather laborious exercise. In your endeavour to arrange admission and institute urgent treatment, you may be inclined to leave much of the associated clerical drudgery incomplete. This tendency may be compounded by the Casualty staff exhorting you to progress to the next patient in the queue of acute cases. However, this results in great inconvenience to houseman and ward-staff alike, for patients eventually arrive on the wards via Casualty with incomplete records or instructions. As a result, the houseman, already outrageously busy in Casualty, is called to the ward by the nursing staff, who require more information regarding the most recent urgent admission before they are able to plan the patient's correct nursing care. It is, then, an economical use of time to ensure that absolutely all paperwork required by the ward-staff (such as case-notes, fluid and drug charts and consent-forms) is completed in the Accident and Emergency Department and accompanies the patient to the ward.

The ability to diagnose conditions unrelated to your own particular speciality and engineer a transfer to the appropriate department is an attribute likely to be highly valued by the senior members of your team. For example, having questioned and examined, in Casualty, a young lady with lower abdominal pain, you might conclude that a diagnosis of pelvic inflammatory disease is likely. This should prompt immediate referral to the on-call gynaecologist; in this way, one can avoid the rigmarole of admission to a surgical ward with subsequent examination by one of your superiors, and, should your diagnosis prove correct, transfer to the gynaecology department. It is important, then, to keep an open mind about possible diagnoses which lie outside your speciality during your initial appraisal of a patient's condition. Even more impressive is the confidence to arrive at a firm conclusion and to have the initiative to take appropriate action. Quite apart from precipitating investigation and treatment of the patient by the correct department, this eases your 'on-take' workload and delights your seniors. However, this skill should be practised with moderation, for over-zealousness may lead to inappropriate requests for 'urgent opinions' from other specialities. The resultant, curt, 'This pain is not of gynaecological origin', for example, from an annoyed and busy gynaecology SHO will do little for your self-esteem and, if repeated too often, may undermine your seniors' confidence in you.

The mechanics of 'routine' transfers are outlined in Chapter 19. One tactic sometimes employed by senior members of your team involves the attempted transfer of a patient who, for some reason, often 'social', stubbornly and unnecessarily remains on your ward. This ploy is sometimes taken to absurd lengths, with batteries of blood tests performed in the hope that some unexpected abnormality might be revealed, thus providing the key to a referral to another speciality. This dubious practice is pathetically unsuccessful, for the motives behind the referral are quite transparent to the potentially 'receiving' teams, who, after all, play a similar game themselves. If possible, you should avoid becoming involved in these futile exercises.

Excuses commonly utilized during housejobs are, by and large, ineffective, being to all but the most imperceptive, tantamount to admissions of guilt or omission. It is most tempting to utter some form of plausible mitigating explanation when one is faced with a manifestly failed practical procedure. For example, gullible patients may easily be convinced that it is quite routine to take blood twice ('one sample from each arm') when, in fact, the initial attempt had missed the target. Some excuses proferred are obviously ridiculous and serve only to compound your apparent incompetence, for example, thrusting, under a nurse's nose, a 'failed' intravenous cannula, mangled by being forced through tissue rather than vein, and, with a disgusted gesture towards its bent tip, exclaiming 'No wonder it wouldn't go in'! Undoubtedly, in these situations, humble honesty is the best policy and is an attribute much respected by nursing staff and patients alike.

An unpleasant sensation which becomes familiar to most housemen is that experienced when your boss demands from you the result of an investigation which you had not yet even instigated. The truth is recommended in this situation but the consequences too awful for

Excuses and Ruses

some to contemplate, and, therefore, various excuses have been invented. Some, in order of credibility, are described below:

'The laboratory machines are currently being serviced and there is an extra delay on all but urgent samples.' This can, in fact, be a genuine excuse (up to twice per year).

'I 'phoned the laboratory this morning and they have no record of having received the sample.' This should be accompanied by a suitable 'look' and gesture intended to convey disgust towards whoever—porters, laboratory staff, in fact anyone except yourself—might be responsible.

'I sent the sample, but, I'm afraid, in the wrong bottle.' While this confirms your status as an idiot, it at least implies that you are a diligent one.

'Oh yes... I asked the medical student to take blood from Mr X.'

The final example illustrates all that is wrong with many excuses. It is a lie; it attempts to shift blame elsewhere and it indicates a shirking of responsibility. Blaming your medical student, particularly when he is not present to protest his innocence, is a vile and odious practice. Houseman and student should exist in a healthy symbiosis. The junior doctor can, given time, instruct his 'shadow', with particular reference to practical skills and ward knowledge; the clinical student, for his part, can assist in various aspects of the houseman's work, simultaneously acquiring confidence and experience in these tasks. In addition, a medical student can act as a houseman's representative when the latter is, literally, required in two places at once. For example, during a 'take' day, the presence of the admitting junior doctor, busy on the consultant's ward-round, might be requested to assess a patient in Casualty. In this situation, provided the potential admission does not constitute an 'emergency', the student could reasonably be asked to perform the initial clerking, thus enabling the houseman to continue with the ward round and quelling the rising impatience of the Casualty staff.

Another common scenario requiring some form of excuse occurs when you are late for your Chief's major ward round. Most Consultants are very reasonable and understanding, and a breathless gallop, tortured expression to convey your current workload and lack of sleep, and a mumbled apology will usually suffice. The 'death warmed up' appearance, described in Chapter 11, is useful in these circumstances.

Arriving late on the ward from home, first thing in the morning, is a different problem, and rather more difficult to justify. Profuse apologies interspersed with jocular comments about your car's unreliability usually work well with Consultants, for most have a penchant for all things automobilian. To placate Ward Sister, you merely have to work twice as hard as usual (and be noticed doing so) for the first hour or two.

The perfect ruse is that which is beneficial to nursing staff, doctor and patient alike. Few such exist, and those that do are often quite specific to a particular speciality. Thus, the most useful 'tricks of the trade' are those that are inherited from your predecessor and which demonstrate anticipation of potential clinical problems. They should be cherished, polished, and, in turn, passed on to your successor. Their selective use, combined with diligence and forethought, should render most excuses redundant.

II
Insomnia

Occasional states of sleeplessness, or perceptions of sleeplessness, are so common as to be considered part of normal experience. However, when such a situation becomes increasingly frequent, or causes distress to the patient, it should be viewed as abnormal, and thus requires evaluation—and, occasionally, treatment. Estimates of the prevalence of sleeplessness in hospital show considerable variation, depending on the definition of insomnia that is used, but rates of approximately 20–30% are common. Therefore, you will frequently be presented the problem of a patient who wants 'something to be done' about his perceived sleeplessness: ironically, to such an extent that it may cause the same problem in yourself.

Many people appear to have unrealistic ideas about the amount of sleep they require, for example, they often do not know that length of sleep becomes shorter in middle and late life. Patients frequently take afternoon 'naps', often through boredom, a common consequence of hospital admission, and still expect that, Morpheus-like, you will magically bestow the gift of 8 hours sleep per night, and thus complain bitterly when you fail to fulfil these expectations.

Insomnia is often secondary to other disorders, notably painful physical conditions (including the discomfort of a full bladder), depressive illness, and anxiety. In addition, causes such as cough, dyspnoea and pruritis are not uncommon. The most frequent cause, in our belief, is *noise*; we are strong advocates of ear plugs. Approximately 15% of patients who complain of sleeplessness will be found to have 'primary' insomnia, in which no cause can be found; resist the temptation to dismiss their complaint, there can be nothing more exasperating to a patient than persistent troublesome sleeplessness, when faced with a disbelieving and unsympathetic houseman.

Evaluation of insomnia includes eliciting its pattern (e.g. initial, middle, or late insomnia), and ascertaining possible causes: do not forget to enquire into excessive caffeine or alcohol consumption (sleep is often disturbed for several weeks after heavy drinking).

'Secondary' insomnia should be alleviated by treatment of the underlying condition. When no cause can be found, encourage regular sleeping habits and discourage night-time coffee and alcohol consumption (you will be surprised how common the latter is within hospitals). In these circumstances, with the failure of simple measures, it is justifiable to prescribe a hypnotic drug, providing there are no contraindications, for a limited period. However, demands for long-term administration should be resisted: reports of addiction, with the development of tolerance and dependence, and producing distressing rebound insomnia upon withdrawal (e.g. on leaving hospital) are increasingly common, as is evidence for impaired daytime performance and possible *permanent* cerebral dysfunction.

Theoretical aspects aside, the choice of hypnotic is probably governed by the patient's need, consultant and nursing staff preference, and recent visits from drug representatives. Generally, it is best to avoid benzodiazepines in the elderly, as these may induce night-time disorientation which you will be called to evaluate. It is best to use short-acting benzodiazepines in order to prevent morning 'hangovers'.

The routine prescription of hypnotics on the 'as required' section of the drug chart is the subject of some controversy. These drugs are most effective in short courses for the acutely distressed patient, and, as mentioned, knowledge of deleterious consequences of continuous use is ever-increasing: nevertheless, such prescription is so common as to invite enquiry when not performed. As in all such matters, it is up to you to decide—balancing adverse effects on one side, against convenience for yourself and the nursing staff, and relatively immediate relief for the patient on the other. Indiscriminate prescription is foolish: self-righteous refusal to do so is unnecessarily punitive.

Insomnia is a condition viewed as distressing by the patient: a concerned attitude, with appropriate evaluation and treatment can only commend yourself to him. Today's High-Tech Medicine frequently leaves patients bewildered as to the nature of their illness, and sleeplessness is an obvious phenomenon, its relief often eliciting greater thanks than many available treatments for disease.

It is likely that you, too, will be similarly troubled by insomnia during your housejobs—your sleeplessness itself may have a number of causes, the most common of which is the auditory over-stimulation by bleeps, telephone calls and alarm clocks. Whilst on duty, nothing is more likely to reduce your duration of sleep than failure to perform a late evening 'round'—all manner of unfortunate events occur in the small hours, many of which can be anticipated. Specifically, make sure drips are working and fluid regimes prescribed, and that instructions are given to the nursing staff as to what action is required in certain eventualities, for example relative hypoglycaemia in a patient on an insulin infusion pump.

You may often feel exasperated about certain apparently unnecessary nocturnal calls from the ward: in our experience, it is better to perform the required task with a wry smile, and return as soon as possible to your bed; rage-induced apoplexy is unlikely to facilitate a quick return to the land of Nod, and can cause disproportionate doctor/nurse friction when the event is recounted during 'morning report'. After the first few weeks, it will often be possible to give instructions by telephone; this does depend on the goodwill of the nurses, so cultivate this from your first day.

Of the many situations requiring your awakening, the majority will be proved necessary. Occasionally, however, you may be asked to perform a seemingly ridiculous task, such as prescribing a hypnotic to a sleeping patient: this is all part of 'life's rich tapestry', and should be pointedly savoured. Other tasks may include certifying death (see Chapter 7) and being called to see the unfortunate patient who has recently cascaded onto the floor from his bed, performing a neurological and orthopaedic examination, and excluding treatable causes of such a fall. This eventually becomes a familiar routine, possessed of its own particular humour.

Though it is in your interest to sleep as much as required, it is worth cultivating the appearance of 'death warmed-up': such facial contortion is guaranteed to induce sympathy in those around you, and impress upon the consultant how hard you must be working. It is surprising that so little is known of the extent of your duties, even by those who work in close proximity, many labouring under the misapprehension that a night on-call is followed by a day off. It is expedient to politely inform them to the contrary.

12
Legalities

In recent years, through various media channels, the general public has become increasingly well-informed about modern medicine, its scientific basis, capabilities, and ethical dilemmas. Concurrently, much emphasis has, rightly, been placed on consumer protection. As a result, western society now demands more from medicine: not only high technology diagnosis and therapy and improved communication, but also better provision for those who are poorly or inappropriately treated. It is within this framework that the public has become more 'litigation conscious', and, consequently, doctors should possess a basic knowledge of the medicolegal aspects of their work. Areas of particular concern to the houseman are included in this chapter.

Prior to commencing work as a houseman, it is contractually necessary to join one of the Medical Defence Bodies which provide medical indemnity. It is important to realize that advice from your own particular Defence Body is available at any time, day or night, whether the problem seems awesome or trivial. If you are involved in legal action related, in any way, to your work as a houseman, then you must, as a priority, inform your Defence Body, whose advice and instructions should be adhered to strictly; in addition, it is usually prudent to provide the Hospital Administrator with relevant details.

'Consent' is a subject which, medicolegally, can cause junior doctors a great deal of concern. Consent may be implied or expressed. During the clerking of a patient, any form of physical contact, for example, blood pressure recording, could in theory be regarded as an assault without the patient's consent. Clearly, to prevent routine medical examination and investigation from degenerating into a time-consuming farce, most consent is viewed as implicit. Expressed consent may be oral (in which case it may be reinforced by being recorded in the case-notes), or written. Legally, the latter is the most 'concrete' evidence of the patient's agreement to investigation or treatment.

Written consent is regarded as mandatory in certain circumstances:
- for any operation (major or minor)
- for certain investigations—especially 'invasive' tests, e.g. endoscopy or angiography
- for any treatment that carries undue risk (e.g. research).

A word of caution is, however, necessary. Simply securing a patient's signature upon a consent form is not necessarily equivalent to obtaining the patient's *informed* consent. Other criteria must be fulfilled before a consent form could be held legally valid. The signature of the patient should be obtained, if possible, in a calm situation, without unavoidable stress; thus, it is inappropriate to thrust pen and form in front of an anxious patient being wheeled down the corridor towards theatre for his elective operation. In addition, the doctor should explain the 'nature and purpose' of the proposed procedure, including details of possible operative and post-operative complications. This is an extremely delicate area, the junior doctor treading a careful, but precarious, line between worrying the patient unnecessarily, and leaving the surgeon open to possible action for subsequent damages. In summary, then, a consent form is used to improve communication, enables the patient to accept or refuse treatment, and provides evidence of consent to a procedure being performed with due 'care and formality'.

In an emergency, where urgent intervention is essential to preserve the life or health of a patient, the requirement for consent may be waived if the patient is unable to give it, as might occur, for example, in the unconscious or mentally disturbed, or in a child. Ideally, the situation should be discussed, and consent obtained, if possible, from a relative or 'responsible' person, although the time involved should not be allowed to jeopardize the patient's well-being.

House surgeons will often be involved in the treatment of children. If an operation is contemplated on a child less than 16 years of age, then, except in an emergency, the written consent of the parents or legal guardian should be obtained (although, interestingly, the law does not actually preclude a child of this age consenting to treatment himself, provided that he can understand the procedure involved and

Legalities

its implications). This is an important practical point: in these cases, consent should be obtained as early as possible if surgical intervention seems a possibility—otherwise, the parents might subsequently be unavailable when you require them to sign the consent form.

Issues regarding consent for sterilization, abortion, and other 'special cases' are usually the province of senior house officers working in a particular speciality, and will not be considered further here.

Occasionally, as a junior doctor, you will be asked by a 'third party' to provide information about a patient who has been under your consultant's care. Typically, these inquiries are conducted over the telephone, and can range from the simple (e.g. a patient's wife inquiring about her husband's post-operative condition) to the rather more complex (e.g. the police investigating a potential crime). Before any information is divulged over the telephone, it is essential that you identify, as far as possible, the identity of the caller. It is far better, for all concerned, that details of patient welfare are discussed in person, and therefore, information provided over the telephone should be brief and of an appropriately broad nature. Whenever you are approached for news of a patient's diagnosis, prognosis, or treatment, confidentiality should be at the forefront of your mind. Unless you have obtained written permission from the individual in question, then the provision of details of his illness to any third party constitutes an invasion of privacy. Naturally, this dogma, in the practical world, is open to interpretation, and the degree of information you would be prepared to discuss with a spouse would differ from that you would impart to another interested party, such as the Press. Nonetheless, in every case, the wishes of the patient should be respected as far as possible: this may result in information being deliberately withheld from relatives or spouses. This undesirable situation should be persistently reviewed with ample time allowed for discussion between doctors, patients and relatives; more often than not, the circumstances resolve naturally and painlessly. It should be noted, however, that confidentiality is an ethical rather than a legal duty. Thus, it is not illegal to disclose details of a patient's illness (although it may be 'morally incorrect'), and, indeed, a court of law can compel a doctor so to do.

Rarely, you may be involved in the treatment of a patient who, you have reason to believe, has been implicated in some form of crime. When police inquiries are not spontaneously forthcoming, you are faced with the dilemma of whether or not to take the initiative by informing the appropriate authorities of your suspicions. Certainly, there is no legal obligation to report a 'petty' crime. If you feel, then, that your knowledge should remain confidential, you would be in no danger of legal action. However, if the crime in question is of a serious nature (e.g. murder, rape or arson) there is a citizen's duty to the community to report it. Between these two extremes, the occasional conflict between the law and the confidentiality ethic must be resolved, using your conscience as guide in each case.

Inquiries from the Press cause less moral agony in house officers, as it is usually recommended that they are immediately referred to the hospital administrator.

'Negligence' is a word which tends to induce palpitations and a frantic verification of Defence Body subscriptions in many doctors. It is reassuring to realize that doctors are not regarded as infallible, and mistakes which do occur are not, of course, automatically regarded as 'negligence'. No matter what disaster befalls you, as long as you acted with reasonable care and skill appropriate in the particular situation—following the 'accepted' practice of the medical profession at that time—then you cannot be found guilty of negligence. Two areas which often produce problems are:

1 Drug administration—errors here are depressingly common and involve the wrong drug, patient, dose, or route. They may be avoided by adopting a pedantic and meticulous policy when administering drugs.

2 Communication—all too often, there is a gross lack of communication between doctors, particularly during the 'hand-over', when the duty doctor assumes the responsibility for any patients with whom he is completely unfamiliar. To provide adequate information in the event of some clinical problem, the relevant case-notes must be kept up-to-date. In addition, the intended management plan of seriously

Legalities

ill or 'at risk' patients should be made perfectly clear to the 'covering' doctor.

Details outlining the medicolegal aspects of the coroner's or law courts are beyond the scope of this book and may be found elsewhere; notes on death certification are detailed in Chapter 7. The diligent and fortunate rarely encounter serious medicolegal difficulty during the pre-registration year. Any real difficulties should be discussed immediately with your seniors, and the advice of your medical defence body should always be sought without hesitation.

13
Nursing Hierarchy

As a medical student, acquaintance with the nursing staff is formally initiated during the 'clinical' period of training, but, often, it is not until the pre-registration year that the need really arises to establish an amicable and knowledgeable rapport with the ward and its members.

The nursing team usually includes the following:

1 Auxiliary nurses—auxiliary nurses, usually recognized by a beige or brown uniform, act as assistants to the trained staff, giving care alone if the patient's needs are few and when simple unmodified tasks are all that is required. Nursing observations of temperature, pulse, blood pressure and respiration are not usually taken by nursing auxiliaries as they are not trained to judge or interpret results.

2 Pupil nurses—pupil nurses are involved in 2 years of training to become 'state enrolled'. The shortened training includes less theoretical input than that of student training (see below). They may be identified by the colour of uniform, belt, or hat-stripe, the 'key' colour usually being green.

3 Student nurses—student nurses undertake 3 years of training to become registered general nurses (staff nurses). Order of seniority, i.e. first, second, or third year students, may be differentiated by the number of stripes on the hat or by belt colour. Unfortunately, there is no strict guideline with uniform as this varies between health authorities and hospitals. As a general rule, that which is green upon a pupil nurse is blue upon a student nurse.

Pupils and students are allocated individual patients to care for along the guidelines of the 'Nursing Process' (see any recent nursing text) and may be of help to the houseman by relaying information about the patient's condition or background. Changes in patient status are referred to a senior nurse (enrolled or registered) so that the appropriate action may be taken. Written daily reports of patients' progress, together with other essential information (such as addresses and telephone numbers of next-of-kin) may be found in the nursing 'Kardex'.

4 Qualified nurses—qualified nurses may be 'enrolled' (SEN or EN) or 'registered' (SRN/RGN or 'staff nurse'). They are usually only distinguished by the SEN or SRN prefix on their name badge, or by the colour of the latter (blue for SRN, green for SEN).

Both enrolled and registered nurses are involved in safe, skilled practical nursing care, day to day ward administration and hospital/community communication. According to their defined roles, registered nurses should, generally, assume the greater responsibility in ward work. For example, recognizing a change in a patient's condition (e.g. as evidenced by wayward nursing observations) should be well within the capabilities of an enrolled nurse, who should then pass on the relevant information to a registered nurse (or, in an emergency, to a doctor). Theoretically, the role of the SRN is, then, to appreciate the significance of this information and take any necessary action.

Naturally, the distinction between these degrees of responsibility blurs very much in practice, and the roles of enrolled and registered nurses are usually interchangeable in terms of ward management. Thus, you may find experienced senior enrolled nurses in charge in the absence of a registered nurse or in the presence of a newly qualified or junior registered nurse. Both SENs and SRNs are familiar with the ward environment and cupboard contents and can point you in the right direction when looking for equipment or information.

It should be noted that 'pupil nurse' status is being phased out, all nurses now being trained towards the 'RGN' qualification. Existing enrolled nurses may remain as SEN or may convert to the higher qualification via extra training.

5 'Extended Role' nursing—handling 'controlled drugs' (or the keys which guard them) is the concern of the registered nurse. However, the enrolled nurse may handle controlled drugs after passing a certificate of competency. Administration of intravenous drugs and additives is usually only performed by staff nurses after attending an intravenous

study course. It is usual nursing policy for the doctor to give the first dose of any intravenous drug (see Chapter 16). Some staff nurses may be trained in phlebotomy and many will perform ECGs when required. Thus, your overall workload may ultimately be decreased if you familiarize yourself with the talents of the nursing staff with whom you work.

6 Ward Sister (male equivalent = Charge Nurse)—the ward sister is in charge of a ward or section and is responsible for the immediate care of patients. She organizes her ward in the manner considered best for those patients, but within the policies laid down by the appropriate Health Authority. She provides overall supervision and guidance and is responsible for student teaching, continued education of her staff, the organization of off-duty rotas and disciplinary action. In the case of a drug error being made by a member of the nursing staff, the event is reported to sister and the junior doctor on call, and any further action then taken if necessary. A good relationship which embraces humour, understanding, trust and mutual respect between houseman and ward sister is vital for the painless and efficient running of the ward and should be cultivated from the outset.

7 Nursing Officers (Clinical Nurse Managers) and Senior Nursing Officers—a group of wards of the same, or similar, speciality, or a department, is controlled by a Unit Nursing Officer. She is well versed in the particular speciality and is responsible for the smooth running of the Unit and for the standard of nursing care. It is the nursing officer who ensures that ward staffing levels are adequate and, in the event of sickness, it is usually she who organizes replacement or extra staff. In these circumstances, you may come into contact with agency staff (qualified nurses employed by a nursing agency). The Senior Nursing Officer co-ordinates the nursing services in an area (often related to one large or a group of small hospitals). With the nursing officers, she plans the objectives and their achievement and keeps top management informed of progress.

8 Principal and Chief Nursing Officers—these comprise top management. However, for the houseman, contact at this level is somewhat unlikely.

14
Nutrition

Nutrition, and its importance in patient management, is a subject with a tendency to be inadequately taught in clinical undergraduate courses, and is frequently passed over whilst discussing patients on ward rounds. It is quite possible, therefore, that the first few weeks of your housejobs will reveal quite astonishing lacunae in your knowledge: these are not only embarrassing, but also deleterious to patient welfare. The hospital in which you work may be fortunate in having a dynamic dietetics department or metabolic unit, with a 'total parenteral nutrition team'. Alternatively, it may not be so lucky, with consequently greater degrees of knowledge being required on your part.

It is probably true that the majority of your patients, on both medical and surgical wards, will not require any specific nutritional intervention. Nevertheless, it is important, when admitting patients, to assess their nutritional status, considering the quality of food that is consumed (not forgetting enquiry as to the consumption of alcohol) and ascertaining whether there has been excess energy output, as occurs, for example, in wasting diseases, prolonged febrile illnesses, vomiting and diarrhoea. The patient will be weighed by the nursing staff. It is occasionally recommended that further evaluation occur, through careful palpation of skin-fold thickness, and assessment of the bulk of the skeletal musculature: this is unlikely to yield much useful information unless there is a doctor with a specific interest in nutrition involved. However, it will doubtless cause a fair amount of bemusement, if not amusement, to all concerned.

Your main involvement in the nutritional management of patients not requiring special dietary consideration will be two-fold. Firstly, as a representative of the hospital, you will doubtless, on occasion, be unfairly castigated for failing to produce an adequate meal: it is prudent, if such complaints persist, to direct them towards catering administration. Secondly, patients will frequently, meekly, request that they might have food brought in by their loved ones. This may fulfil psychological needs and should not be resisted, providing there is no contraindication. It is worth remembering, however, that such food parcels might contain alcoholic beverages: ward policy or patient welfare may preclude such provision.

Many of your patients, however, will require further dietary consideration. Special diets include those not only governed by religious or ethical persuasion, but also those determined by medical necessity, as occurs, for example, in the diets of those suffering from obesity, diabetes mellitus, dysphagia, those with liver or renal failure, the jaundiced, and those receiving monoamine oxidase inhibitors. The theoretical content of these diets is governed by knowledge of aberrant metabolic pathways, the practical administration being effected by the ward dietitian. Such diets are commonly prepared. Again, you are unlikely to be extensively involved, apart from recognizing the need for a special diet and realizing that the meals are likely to be unflavoursome for the patient, who will thus require greater degrees of psychological titillation.

Before one can discuss the specifics of nutritional supplementation, the diagnosis of malnutrition has to be made. The most common problem here stems from the 'talking heads' ward round. This is the situation where doctors congregate around the bed and talk to the patient's head, the rest of him being covered by the bedclothes. The simple matter of withdrawing the bedclothes and seeing the wasted body of the patient will make the diagnosis of malnutrition. This circumstance illustrates how good communication with members of the nursing staff may pay dividends.

Degrees of protein energy malnutrition are common amongst surgical patients, diagnosed when weighing of the patient reveals more than 15% of body weight to have been lost: this has effects upon the rehabilitation of the patient, since the immune system is less able to resist infection, wounds take longer to heal, and the return home is consequently delayed. Such malnutrition can be confirmed by tests of liver function (and palpation of skeletal musculature): if weight loss

Nutrition

greater than 15% occurs, and plasma albumin concentration is less than 30 g/l, urgent nutritional intervention is required, usually through nasogastric or parenteral feeding. However, most such situations should ideally be anticipated and prevented by appropriate therapy in the first place.

It is worth noting here that short-term changes in body weight are often the result of changes in the body fluid compartments, therefore always assess cardiovascular status and fluid balance prior to committing a patient to hyperalimentation.

Nasogastric, or orogastric, feeding involves the instillation of a fine bore tube into the stomach lumen, via the appropriate orifice, with intermittent or continuous infusion of liquid feed, the volume and contents of which are normally specified on the bottle, and charted at the end of the patient's bed: it is occasionally necessary to specify the regimen on the patient's prescription sheet. Very often an intermittent feed will lead to troublesome diarrhoea and many people now favour continuous infusion. Quite apart from requiring a large degree of support (it is difficult to preserve self-esteem with a nasogastric tube *in situ*), these patients will require daily weighing, accurate fluid assessment charts, and initially at least, daily estimation of serum urea and electrolytes. It is unlikely, therefore, that your appearance at the bedside, armed with a syringe and needle, will be received with joy. In rare circumstances where a patient has undergone a surgical procedure, a feeding jejunostomy or gastrostomy tube may be *in situ*. The principles of feeding are the same as nasogastric tubes but care must be taken of the catheter entry site.

Further steps into control of patients' nutritional welfare include parenteral feeding, this occurring when enteral feeding is not possible, nutrients usually being delivered via a catheter inserted in the subclavian vein or external or internal jugular vein and thence into the superior vena cava. It is important to be aware of the complications of insertion of such a line (e.g. pneumothorax, or nerve damage), therefore a chest X-ray and examination must follow this. It is important to know that this line is used for nutrition only; it will require replacement if used for other reasons as septicaemia may ensue. Therefore if measurement of central venous pressure is required, a separate line must be used, and a peripheral line inserted should the patient require intravenous antibiotics, blood transfusion, or other fluids. Great care must be taken to avoid line sepsis and there will almost certainly be a protocol for dressing of the line entry site.

An impressive array of total parenteral nutrition (TPN) fluids are in existence. They are generally dispensed in 3-litre bags prepared in the Pharmacy. The content of the nutrient solution and additives is determined by daily monitoring. Patients receiving TPN are commonly, in large hospitals at least, assessed by a 'nutrition team', consisting of a gastroenterologist, chemical pathologist, pharmacist, and dietitian. This team will require that the patient be weighed daily, have his fluid balance accurately assessed (often necessitating bladder catheterization), and be subjected to daily venesection for urea and electrolytes ('U & Es'), serum glucose, and tests of hepatic function. Patients undergoing such management thus need reassurance that they are not merely the connecting piece to a convoluted system of tubes and wires. It behoves the nursing and medical staff to consider needs other than the recording of information. One must also be aware that a patient receiving parenteral nutrition may be losing the equivalent of 140 ml of blood per week via repeated sampling. Ensure that only the minimum amount of blood is removed and keep a careful watch on the patient's haemoglobin—they may need a transfusion from the blood lost due to analysis!

In patients who have been receiving nutritional supplementation, whatever the route, secondary anorexia is a problem: by the time nutritional supplementation is withdrawn, the desire to eat has disappeared and much encouragement is required. Various ploys have been adopted, but providing the patient with boiled sweets and enticing foodstuffs early in the resumption of normal diet often prevents this troublesome complication.

Patients suffering from malignant disease require special consideration. The loss of appetite and weight that is associated with disseminated carcinoma is troublesome to patient and carers alike; it is found that judicious use of alcoholic beverages, such as sherry, can be helpful as an appetite stimulant. Strict adherance to diets in the terminally ill is often considered to be inappropriate; far better that the patient acutally enjoy food in his last few days, provided, that is, that symptoms produced by consuming an inappropriate diet do not overshadow that enjoyment.

Finally, some words of advice. During the year of your housejobs, the hours that you will work will be longer, and more irregular, than those to which you have been accustomed. It is tempting to avoid meals, when the pressure of work is particularly great, in the belief that your physical presence on the wards is the most important factor in patient welfare. It is not. Avoid these rescue fantasies. The most important factor is *your* physical and mental health. Hypoglycaemia-induced fainting whilst running to a cardiac arrest is unlikely to be welcomed by the patient.

15
Peripheral Staff

There exists an increasing tendency for the development of a truly multi-disciplinary approach to patient care in general hospital medicine and surgery. This welcome change represents, partially, a return to an holistic approach, though, unlike pre-technological medicine, where the various aspects of care usually arose from individual endeavour, today's 'care' is likely to stem from a number of individuals, each responsible for their chosen area of speciality, all parts functioning under the direction of the supervising consultant.

As a houseman, therefore, you are likely to participate with other members of staff, all working for the perceived 'good' of a patient. Staff disparagingly designated as 'peripheral' during one's undergraduate training acquire a central importance in the ward management of many medical and surgical conditions. For example, your involvement in the care of a patient recovering from a cerebro-vascular accident will involve elucidation of cause (where possible or appropriate), instigation of measures designed to prevent its repetition, anticipation and prevention of complications, encouragement, and education. Valuable though these measures undoubtedly are, the patient would be unlikely to have a successful rehabilitation without the involvement of physiotherapists to maximize potential mobility; speech therapists to attempt correction of dysphasia and dysarthria, if present; occupational therapists to restore fine muscle function and gradually readapt the patient to his own home; and social workers to organize the provision of social service resources.

Furthermore, such multiplicity of input from paramedical staff is in itself probably insufficient, without support, advice, and assistance from other hospital staff whose role may not have a recognized clinical component, but who nevertheless are essential to the patient: domestics, porters, and canteen staff are obvious examples.

Studies frequently reveal that it is neither doctors nor nurses who have the greatest patient contact, such accolades usually being given to ward domestic staff: experience indicates that the individual most craved by patients, however, is neither medical, nor paramedical, nor ancillary—but instead that person who embodies life 'outside', namely the paperman. For it is he who provides the news, gossip, confectionery, and, regrettably, cigarettes, the four commodities most desired by the majority of patients, ward morale being rarely so low as when the paperman has unexpectedly failed to appear.

Quite apart from ensuring best possible patient care, involvement of paramedical staff is of great help to you, by allowing delegation of activity, if not responsibility. Physiotherapists, for example, will perform lung function tests if asked nicely (and if indicated): ultrasonographers may perform Doppler assessment of the peripheral pulses: ECG technicians organize cardiac ultrasound and 24-hour recording. These examples indicate that the paramedical staff's capabilities exceed their perceived initial attributes. Similarly, dietiticians and pharmacy staff, by the provision of patient advice sheets, relieve some of the responsibility for patient education from yourself: *their* advice to *you* is occasionally life-saving. Your workload can therefore be diminished substantially without inordinately increasing that of your colleagues.

It would be narrow-minded to assume that such alleviation of pressure of work on the houseman is only possible with the aid of paramedical staff; ward clerks, appointment staff, and your consultants' secretaries may take on many of the logistical responsibilities such as ordering of investigations, filing of results, and correspondence with medical colleagues.

One's year as a houseman is characterized by its unpredictability: niceties such as regular ingestion of food, evacuation of body waste-products and prolonged ablution are likely to be disturbed by one's bleep. It is therefore crucial to be in the good books of the switchboard staff, who may, on persuasion, 'sift' through one's calls, when requested, to ensure that your weekly bath isn't disturbed, for example, by a feckless technician informing you that a bottle has been incompletely labelled. It is easy to become charming when the rewards are so great.

16
Practical Dilemmas and their Resolution

Frequently, during your year as a houseman, you will find your skill, or luck, in performing practical procedures stretched to its limit. There inevitably comes a time when the crimson of your embarrassed face matches the stain on the bedclothes when, for example, having taken five attempts at venepuncture, you eventually succeed but then, in an effort to attain a good sample, pull the plunger out of the end of the syringe. Fear not. Disasters happen to us all. Happily, they usually injure our pride rather than the patient.

The Chapter aims to pinpoint and facilitate those procedures which most commonly cause us sympathetic overactivity and, occasionally, a desire for a change of career.

Intravenous cannulation

A variable degree of expertise in this field is usually attained as a medical student. However, it is one thing to achieve a 20% success rate when any success is an unexpected bonus, and quite another when you have four cannulae to insert in difficult patients on a busy ward with the Consultant's round looming and your bleep chirping persistently.

Inevitably, the chances of first time success with an intravenous cannulation are inversely proportional to the urgency of that particular procedure. Thus, if you absolutely *have* to secure a drip in a fat diabetic patient possessing a single accessible vein minutes before he is due in theatre, then, of course, you will be unable to do so. In other words, your confidence and attitude are probably as important as anything else; conscious efforts to remain unhurried, calm and methodical may pay unexpected dividends. Conversely, if you *are* a genuine incompetent, then this tactic serves merely to make you look not only bumbling but also slow.

Rule two regarding intravenous cannulation involves a reassessment of the need for the cannula: if you can reasonably avoid resiting a drip, then do so. It is amazing how often an intravenous infusion is discontinued at precisely the time the cannula 'tissues'.

Having established the requirement for intravenous cannulation, the following points may be useful to consider:

1 Everyone, even an anaesthetist, is 'beaten' by a lack of veins at some stage in their career. Therefore, do not interpret failure as a direct insult to your ability. It follows that it is logical to limit yourself to a specific number of attempts: five is arbitrarily regarded as a maximum. Any more than this is unkind and leaves the patient looking as though he has just been in a road accident (which, indeed, might be the case). In addition, after attempt number six, your nerves are likely to be so hopelessly shredded that simply managing to insert the cannula into the patient's arm, regardless of any veins, should be interpreted as 'success'.

2 Do not hurry proceedings; instead, wait patiently until a suitable vein appears. Traditional methods of coaxing shy veins into a visible or palpable state include slapping the patient's arm, letting the arm hang in a dependent position over the side of the bed and immersing the limb in warm water for 5 minutes. Shaving the appropriate area sometimes aids the search for veins and is appreciated by nurses and patients alike: most of the pain associated with intravenous cannulae is actually caused by their removal, when hairs are agonizingly plucked out as the adhesive plaster is peeled away.

3 If the 'usual' sites are unavailing, it is justifiable to attempt to cannulate veins in less ideal areas (especially if, for example, the patient is having a drip for a very short period), e.g. antecubital fossa or dorsum of hand. Similarly, if particularly miniscule veins are the only vessels on offer, then a much smaller cannula should be considered (if this is a practical possibility, for blood transfusions will easily clog if administered through a cannula of small lumen).

4 Regardless of your technical expertise and persistence, you will occasionally be faced with a multiple punctured but dripless patient. At this stage, it is wise to at least call upon the experience and skill

of your superior, or, perhaps more reasonably, the duty anaesthetist. An anaesthetist defeated by peripheral veins will suggest 'central-lines' or 'cut-downs', both subjects outside the scope of this book.

Venesection

Again, the problem with this procedure lies in locating a suitable vein and therefore the techniques described above should be employed in difficult cases.

It is always wise to consider carefully the laboratory tests indicated immediately prior to taking blood from a patient. Are there any analyses which are likely to be required soon but which could just as easily be derived from the sample you are about to take? This foresight might save you work and the patient further puncture-wounds; for example, taking a sample of adequate volume to allow 'Group and Saving' (in addition to the full blood count), when a transfusion is anticipated, is sensible practice, (see Chapter 4).

When the patient's peripheral veins prove refractory to your coaxing, a venous sample may be readily obtained (especially in an emergency, for example in a shocked patient) by a 'femoral stab'. This involves the removal of blood from the femoral vein, the needle being inserted 2 cm medial to the palpable femoral pulse.

Urinary catheters

The insertion of a urinary catheter is usually a straightforward procedure. Clumsiness is the most common problem, resulting in the lubricating jelly covering not only the catheter but also the doctor's sterile gloves and much of the bed. In this situation, attempts to gently insert the catheter prove ineffectual and the remedy lies in making a completely fresh start.

Prior to catheter insertion, the retaining balloon should be checked to ensure that it inflates properly. This is best carried out while you are waiting for the lignocaine gel to take effect. Often, the catheter meets resistance, particularly as it passes through the prostatic urethra.

This can be overcome by gentle, controlled pressure, which may insinuate the catheter through the narrow lumen. Alternatively, repeated slight withdrawals followed by attempts at reintroduction may be successful. Paradoxically, the procedure can be facilitated by using a catheter of larger bore, probably because the increased size renders it less flexible. It should be stressed that unsuccessful catheterization, after reasonable efforts as outlined above, should be abandoned for fear of damage to the patient's urethra, and assistance sought from your superiors. Any discomfort voiced by the patient as you attempt to inflate the catheter balloon should make you suspect that the balloon is in the urethra rather than the bladder, in which case, the catheter should be introduced further or the procedure postponed.

There is a common fallacy that leakage around an established catheter implies that a catheter of larger bore should be employed. This is usually untrue. Such leakage is commonly caused by a blocked catheter or bladder 'irritability', and appropriate therapy (bladder washouts, antibiotics for infection or bladder relaxant medication) instituted. Sometimes, the problem may be miraculously solved by withdrawing a little fluid from the retaining balloon (an over-inflated balloon can be very irritating to a bladder).

Refusal of the catheter balloon to deflate when removal of the device is required is rather alarming to doctor and patient alike, but not at all uncommon. The problem may be solved by overinflating the balloon until it bursts; the patient should be warned of the impending, very audible, 'pop', otherwise he may fear that his bladder has exploded. If this trick fails, then the instillation of tiny amounts of certain solvents into the balloon results in instant success but should not be attempted without the advice of your seniors.

Arterial puncture

Sites from which arterial blood is usually taken are, in order of frequency, the radial, femoral and brachial arteries. The actual technique is a rather personal matter, and competence and confidence evolve naturally quite rapidly with experience. Points to note include:
1 The biochemistry laboratory should be warned of the sample's im-

minent arrival if you are fortunate enough not to have to perform the analysis yourself.

2 Prior to removing blood from the radial artery, the patency of the ulnar artery should be tested.

3 The procedure is painful and often warrants a local anaesthetic infiltration (especially when using the femoral route).

4 The syringe (and, if necessary, 'butterfly') must be flushed through with heparin before use, otherwise the wrath of the biochemistry department will be upon you (not to mention a large bill for damaged analytical equipment).

5 Ensure that all air bubbles, which might otherwise invalidate the results obtained, are evacuated from the sample.

6 Press hard via a gauze pad over the puncture site for a full 5 minutes to prevent haematoma formation.

7 The sample obtained should be placed in a bag, with ice, and transported to the laboratory immediately. Thus, another pair of hands should be readily available either to act as porter or to prevent bleeding as outlined in 6.

8 Occasionally, you may be uncertain as to whether the sample obtained is arterial or venous. The definitive test involves withdrawing a venous sample in the usual way, using a heparinized syringe, and performing blood gas analysis on both 'arterial' and venous specimens. If the results are identical, then, obviously, you have failed to obtain a true arterial sample and must therefore think of an excuse to puncture the patient again (honesty sometimes works well).

9 It is worthwhile warning the patient that this is an 'unusual' blood test before you attempt the procedure because, being quite accustomed to venepuncture, he may become anxious when you puncture an unusual site, such as the groin, especially if you appear to have some difficulty with the technique.

Nasogastric tubes

The routine insertion of nasogastric tubes is nearly always performed by the nursing staff; thus, junior doctors, as a rule, know nothing about this procedure. Rather absurdly, in the rare instance of institution of fine-bore nasogastric feeding, most hospitals require that the fine-bore tube is inserted by a doctor. Inevitably, the task falls in your direction and really is very simple: the introducer and tube are both coated with a lubricating jelly, and passed along the floor of the nose. When the patient feels the tube at the back of his throat, he is asked to swallow so that it is guided in the desired direction, down the oesophagus and into the stomach. The introducer is gently removed and the free end of the apparatus is secured, usually by means of a strip of tape, to the patient's forehead (standard nasogastric tubes are, of course, attached to a drainage bag). A chest X-ray is recommended before feeding is commenced, to ensure that the end of the fine-bore tube is situated in the stomach.

Reflex gagging during the procedure can sometimes create difficulties. Repeated withdrawals and reinsertions, with instruction to the patient to breathe through his mouth and to swallow at the appropriate time usually result in success. Alternatively, a pair of forceps may be used to guide the tube in the correct direction when it appears at the back of the throat; a benzocaine lozenge sucked for a few minutes will facilitate this procedure (sucked by the patient, *not* the doctor).

Intravenous drugs

According to hospital policy, you will be called upon to give all, or at least the first dose, of intravenous drugs. This sounds very straightforward but may present technical riddles best solved by seeking the help of the senior nurse on duty until you become more experienced with the technique yourself. In fact, nursing staff must attend certain courses and obtain specific certificates before they are permitted to administer intravenous drugs. Thus, they will undoubtedly be much better informed than you and it is wise to swallow your pride at an early stage in your first housejob and ask someone to demonstrate the basics of drawing up and administering intravenous drugs if such information was not imparted to you as a medical student. Inevitably, it is the practical rather than the theoretical hurdle which causes most junior doctors to hesitate with intravenous drug procedure.

Naturally, the rudiments of the treatment of anaphylactic shock should be firmly imprinted in your brain whenever you give intravenous drugs; never forget to check the patient's name, the drug itself (and its expiry date), the dose and the fact that the patient really is supposed to be receiving that particular therapy. Traditionally, the doctor tends to forget to sign for the administration of the drug in the patient's drug-chart. This omission can lead to dangerous repetition of treatment.

Electrocardiograms

These are highly idiosyncratic machines. Ideally, avoid performing ECGs yourself at all, when practicable, as the procedure is irritatingly time-consuming. The nursing staff, especially in Casualty, often perform ECGs if asked nicely, and you may be fortunate enough to have the services of an 'ECG lady'.

However, in emergencies and 'out of hours', the onus will be on you to operate the machine. Difficulties encountered are frequently frustratingly simple, yet disproportionately insoluble (e.g. the lack of a roll of ECG paper, or the inability of anyone to recall which lead goes to which limb; although, usually, there is a tattered and fading colour-code to be found somewhere on the metal casing of the machine).

The best plan is to become intimate with your particular ECG machine one evening when you are on call and have nothing better to do. A little time spent methodically examining its mixed mass of wires, metal, paper and electrode jelly seems worthwhile when, confronted by an 'arrested' patient, you are expected to slickly set up the machine and rapidly obtain a valid tracing.

Others

Depending on your enthusiasm, expertise and diligence, and the workload of other members of your team, you may be called upon to perform practical procedures other than the more basic ones described in this chapter. These include tapping pleural and peritoneal effusions, aspirating joints, performing lumbar punctures and inserting central venous cannulae and suprapubic catheters. The only realistic advice that might be proferred in such circumstances, within the confines of this book, is to do *nothing* that you are not entirely confident is within your capabilities and, should any problems arise during the procedure, do not hesitate to contact your seniors for help. For further information regarding these 'advanced' techniques, the reader should consult a text of practical procedures (*Procedures in Practice*. Articles from the British Medical Journal (1981) Stephen Lock Ed. The Devonshire Press, is particularly recommended).

17
Priorities

The living take priority over the dead.

18
Private Patients

During your year as a houseman, you may occasionally be responsible for the day-to-day care of your consultants' private patients. This task, which might not contractually be yours, may cause a number of difficult problems, adding to those arising from the management of your National Health Service patients.

The consultants for whom you work may have a thriving private practice, and only rarely be seen on the wards: alternatively, they may eschew the financial rewards and freedom from administrative bureaucracy that private medicine offers, in order to fully commit themselves to the NHS. Obviously, consultants have a right to choose how they should spend their time, providing they fulfil their agreed contractual obligations.

In *your* care of private patients it is prudent to place political, or ethical, considerations to one side, and treat them as you would all other patients. Though conscience may dictate that you refuse to participate in the management of 'PPs', such action would be unlikely to gain the support of your colleagues: the medical profession is essentially conservative, and wishes to avoid controversy. In many respects your future career hinges upon your consultants' references and it would be a pity to jeopardize your livelihood by impetuous decisions made before you were able to exert control over your medical destiny. Besides, the occasional financial remuneration from your consultant, in recognition of your help with private patients, might likely to compromise any ideals that you may have.

Private patients have a propensity to be foreign. This may either make history-taking impossible, save for attempts at salvage involving sign-language, or, if a translator is available, inordinately prolonged. Quite apart from posing communication problems, private patients often tend to arrive unannounced, without medical notes or the results

Private Patients

of essential investigations, on the morning of proposed extensive surgical procedures. You will gradually acquaint yourself with this situation, and indeed, come to expect it.

It must be stated that the vast majority of private patients are affable citizens whose employment offers, as a perk, private health insurance. Such characters cause few difficulties and may seem disproportionately grateful for the care that you offer.

Surgeons appear to have greater numbers of private patients than their medical colleagues, presumably because much of general surgery is undertaken as an elective procedure. Patients in this situation pose a number of problems. Resentment can ride high amongst operating theatre staff who might receive no financial remuneration for their activities, and who may perceive inequality in the preferential addition of 'PPs' to operating lists. Since two consultants are required at the time of operation, one to anaesthetize and one to cut, the exact placement of the patient on the operating list is subject to negotiation. Such high-level consultations frequently occur at midnight of the day before the operation, using the on-call house surgeon as an intermediary.

Private patients often feel themselves entitled to the attention of a particular team: as such, difficulties are encountered when the duty houseman is called to see the private patient of another firm. In this situation, it is appropriate to inform the responsible consultant of any problem that may occur: indeed, as a general rule, always let your consultant know of any unforeseen difficulties arising in his private patients.

Such patients under the care of physicians pose their own set of problems. They have a tendency to arrive on the ward by a circuitous route. It has been known for a successfully resuscitated moribund individual to recover to the extent that the patient informed the attendant team of his desire 'to go private'. It is wise to inform your consultant of these cases as soon as possible—he will be eternally grateful, excellent references being guaranteed.

Similarly, patients occasionally nurse, rightly or wrongly, grievances against those responsible for their care in an NHS capacity, and request that they 'go private'. You may therefore either be the donor, or recipient, of such individuals: these situations seem only rarely to occur in surgical patients.

A final word. When dealing with private patients, always indicate that their consultant is possessed of god-like genius—it's good for their trade, your career, and the patient's peace of mind.

19
Referrals

The increasing tendency to sub-specialize in hospital medicine makes the persistence of 'general' surgeons or physicians ever more unlikely. Obviously, this situation has arisen as a result of the fantastic advances in medical knowledge that have occurred only comparatively recently: it is simply no longer possible to know something of everything. As such, making 'referrals' or requests for specialist advice, now form a significant part of the house officer's work, it being your fate, as most junior member of the firm, to arrange, and less frequently, to receive, referrals. These may be conducted by personal visit, telephone, or by written word.

When referring to a 'centre of excellence', whether this be institution, firm or individual cerebrum, the following points must be considered:

1 Referrals are addressed to the consultant's firm, not to designated individuals. It may be common knowledge that it is the hard-working registrar who is destined to eventually provide the goods; but it is simply bad form to ignore tradition.

2 Administrative details should follow, including the name of your consultant, yourself, and your bleep number; the patient's name, date of birth, and employment; if an outpatient, his address, and that of his general practitioner; if an inpatient, the name of the ward where he or she is currently residing.

3 Clinical information is then presented: features on admission, tentative initial diagnosis, results of investigations, revised diagnosis.

4 Next, and most important, how it is felt the greater knowledge and experience of the agent to whom the referral is addressed might aid in the management of the patient under consideration.

5 Finally, an indication as to whether the patient requires seeing urgently, or more routinely.

A few points require elaboration. If writing a referral form, such communication technically constitutes a letter: as such, you should attempt to observe as many grammatical niceties as your education allows. Like all forms of presentation to senior members of the medical profession, it is best to proceed with the history–examination–investigation–diagnosis framework so endlessly rehearsed whilst a medical student.

It is sensible to anticipate the investigations that might be required by the second doctor. Some of these should be obvious: for example, a cardiologist will be likely to require recent chest X-rays and ECGs, together with results of serial estimations of cardiac enzymes, should these be appropriate.

Avoid the tendency to describe *all* referrals as requiring 'urgent' attention. Though prompt interview by the specialist may increase your kudos, when presenting at the next ward round, such action ultimately denies *urgent* attention when this is truly indicated. Similarly, labelling all your patients as requiring urgent review might lead outsiders to speculate as to the extent of clinical skills residing within your firm.

The intricacies of referral may constitute a tiresome, convoluted process. With practice however, this important area of your job may be rendered considerably less time-consuming. Nevertheless, it is prudent to avoid the referral requests, once considered traditional, that ran as follows:

> Dear Specialist,
>
> re : Patient X
>
> Please see and do the necessary.
>
> Yours, etc.
>
> Dr Non-specialist.

One wonders how often this prompted the informative reply,

> 'Patient seen. Necessary done'

Referrals

In view of your limited knowledge, and minimal experience, it is unlikely that your role in receiving referrals, from fellow hospital doctors, will be anything other than waving the appropriate form at, or passing on messages to, the more senior members of your firm. Therefore, always remember to check your white coat pockets at the end of the day; otherwise, all 'urgent' referrals will become 'routine'.

Hospital policy may dictate that, when 'on-take', it is the houseman who receives external referrals from general practitioners, and other agencies. You can only hope that the quality of referrals that you receive is akin to that of those you deliver.

20
Relatives

Talking to the relatives of your patients is a time-consuming, and often troublesome task: however, with sensitivity, forethought, and average skills of communication, this activity, which often initially appears onerous, is potentially one of the most rewarding areas of your job. Being the most junior member of the consultant's firm, you are the most approachable, to both patient and relative alike: your position as final common pathway in patient management and explanation is thus one of great responsibility. As a student, however, the emphasis on your involvement is on 'clerking' patients: it is likely, therefore, that your undergraduate training will probably have left you inexperienced in talking to relatives about their loved ones' illnesses.

On admission, patients, for a variety of reasons, may be unable to give an adequate history of their complaints. Obviously, this is the case with young children, in whom the reassuring presence of a parent is essential during the first few hours in hospital. Parents will be needed to sign the consent form of all children under the age of 16 years: therefore, when faced with a seemingly endless queue of patients waiting to be admitted, it is prudent to commence with the children, since the parents will be essential to sensible clerking, and may well have other children at home, to whom they are keen to return.

Generally, relatives do not need to be present whilst a history is taken. However, patients may be uncommunicative for a variety of reasons; for example, they may be foreign, deaf, mute, disorientated, prone to confabulation, comatose or dead. On occasion, patients may be plain unwilling to disclose information, maintaining 'There's nothing wrong with me!', despite manifest evidence to the contrary. In the absence of accurate subjective information it seems expedient to enquire elsewhere in an attempt to avoid practising medicine that might otherwise be described as 'veterinary'.

It is sad that although patients usually find it easy to give sufficient information to satisfy the enquirer when describing physical complaints, such detailed information is likely to be less forthcoming when describing symptoms perceived as psychological, or due to loss of social function. Reticence is an understandable phenomenon in those who have become incapacitated by problems such as incontinence, falls, and confusion: relatives may then be the only accurate sources of information. Additionally, a history of noncompliance with medication, drug abuse, and excessive alcohol consumption may similarly become available.

Whilst examining patients, it is generally advisable that relatives are absent from the bedside: this may provide a suitable forum for the revelation of details that the patient had earlier wished to keep concealed. Young children, without exception, and the elderly, on occasion, will benefit from the continued presence of a close relative. Outside of these age groups, reassurance can be made available by the chaperoning abilities of a member of the ward nursing staff. It is worth noting that patients often feel unable to confide in doctors, preferring instead to reveal information of immense importance to the ward nurses, or medical students; always enquire as to whether this has occurred.

After admission, involvement with relatives is likely to be less intense, providing the patient's clinical condition improves. Special care in communication will be required with the relatives of those patients in whom this does not apply (see Chapter 5 and 7). There is, however, a need for continuing liaison with the relatives of patients who are undergoing a prolonged stay in hospital, with extensive investigations (even if the trend is towards recovery), in order to explain *what* is happening, and *why*—recovery does not preclude running commentary! As discharge becomes imminent, relatives will need to be informed of the proposed day of leaving hospital; the necessity of continuing medication, should this be intended; the measure of social support offered; and the date of any outpatient appointments. Further details are given in Chapter 21. When discharge looms, it is important that adequate time is made available, in order to inform patients and relatives what is to be expected in the convalescence, and to explain tell-tale symptoms of relapse, together with appropriate action.

Experience reveals the vast majority of relatives of patients to be caring, kind individuals, loving in their provision of fragments of the patient's domestic environment, eager to impart as much information as is requested, sparing of doctors' time, and grateful to nurses, doctors and other hospital staff. There are those, indeed, in whom such qualities are so pronounced as to render your patient a disservice. It is not uncommon for relatives, in their understandable desire to have their loved ones returned home, to overestimate their potential as care-givers and underestimate the strain that caring for the convalescent or ill might impose, with potentially disastrous results. In these cases, tactful elaboration of the difficulties that might arise, and of possibilities of alternative accommodation (e.g. hospices, Part III sheltered housing and convalescent homes) is likely to reduce overall morbidity in the community. Conversely, it may be the patient who has an unrealistic perception of his abilities. Relatives may then be essential in reinforcing the opinions of the doctors and nurses, whether this be on matters such as admission, treatment plans or after-care.

There is, however, a small minority of individuals, not characterized by the redeeming qualities outlined above. Such relatives may be evasive, or excessively intrusive; negligent, or interfering; critically eloquent, or verbally abusive. Complaint may be justified, and each should be judged on its own merit: on occasion, the impression is that grievances levelled at the carers arise from attempts to assuage the guilt that relatives may experience for having felt, or been deemed, 'inadequate' in the past: this may, or may not, have been the case.

This is not the place for didactic discussion of such psychopathology; instead, some words of advice.

- The houseman is the representative of the consultant—therefore, only inform relatives of confirmed policy decisions, thereby avoiding the trap of 'Well, Doctor X said so-and-so. . .'. Should this approach prove unsatisfactory, advise the discontented relatives to address their complaints to the relevant authority.

Relatives

- Exercise caution in commitment—avoid giving clinical details, prognoses, and discharge plans over the telephone, since these are liable to misinterpretation: it is prudent never to commit yourself in writing (and indeed should never be necessary for a houseman so to do).

- Retain clinical detachment at all times—though a relative, or patient, for that matter, may appear a hatchet-faced old boot it would be unwise to describe them as such.

- It is best to avoid making oneself available to relatives by bleep: advise them that appointments with the medical staff should be arranged through the ward clerk or consultant's secretary.

- Remember, finally, that the bleep is a double-edged weapon: though it may be the bane of your life, it is possible to arrange that your colleagues call you away for an 'emergency', 10 minutes into a meeting with particularly obstreperous relatives.

21
Routes of Exit

The ways in which a patient leaves hospital vary in both mode and ultimate destination. A straightforward discharge to the patient's own home is the most simple and obvious example: this, and other mechanisms whereby a patient leaves your care, are described below.

1 *Death*—see Chapter 7.

2 *Transfer to another hospital*—this situation arises most commonly when you are employed in a 'Regional Centre' of some sort. All patients requiring certain specialist treatment (e.g. radiotherapy) will be referred to your consultant, from a wide catchment area, for the treatment specifically offered by your department. When this treatment is complete (and assuming that the patient is unfit to be discharged directly to his home) the patient is usually transferred back to the hospital from which he was referred. Your role in this manoeuvre is: to anticipate the transfer; contact the receiving hospital to ascertain when, and on which ward, a bed might be available (it should be noted that minimal persuasion should be required to engineer the transfer at the desired time as the onus is on the receiving hospital to fulfil their obligation to reassume the care of the patient after his specialist treatment); ensure that appropriate transport is arranged—many transport departments require 48 hours notice to guarantee that transport will be available where and when required, hence the importance of anticipation. The nursing staff usually take care of these arrangements but they will need to be informed of a planned discharge as soon as possible; write a transfer letter detailing the salient features of the particular case (the receiving medical team, being the one which referred the patient in the first place, should already be familiar with the history and other details and, so, this section of the letter may be kept reasonably brief), the timespan, form and efficacy of the treatment which the patient received under your care, and current medication

(including details of duration of drug regimes where appropriate); ensure that the patient, and his relatives, understand why and when he is being transferred back to his original hospital.

Clearly, this entire situation could be inverted in that a patient under your care on a general medical or surgical ward might require urgent specific treatment at an appropriate Regional Centre. In this case, your immediate superior will probably initiate the transfer, but the task of arranging transport, ensuring that a bed is available, informing the patient and writing a detailed referral letter will inevitably fall in your direction.

3 *Self-discharge*—very rarely, a patient might decide that he wishes to discharge himself from hospital. If this action is at odds with the wishes of the medical team, then this situation comes under the heading of 'leaving hospital against medical advice'.

In most cases, the patient's decision is borne from frustration and confusion regarding his treatment. This invariably arises from a lack of communication on the ward. An unhurried, detailed and sympathetic clarification of the rationale underlying the patient's management, with apologies and explanations for any delays experienced, is often enough to reassure the patient that the best plan is to stay in hospital.

Occasionally you might fully agree with the patient's proposed action, although your opinion might not mirror those of your superiors. This dilemma may be resolved by paying 'lip service' to the 'against medical advice' line.

Even more rarely, having conversed as described above with the patient, you might conclude that he is not of sound mind to make a rational decision. This occurs most obviously with the acutely confused patient (e.g. post-operatively) in which case, a deaf ear and appropriate sedative are usually employed, with a subsequent search for the cause of the confusional state. However, other examples of possible mental disorder apparently influencing a patient's decision to discharge himself may be less clear-cut and this is the time to seek advice from another member of your medical team or from a psychiatrist.

If the patient is clearly thinking rationally, has accepted and understood your balanced remonstrations, and yet persists with his wish for discharge, then the procedure is as follows:

(i) Decide whether or not you need to inform your superior. In practice, he is generally able to add little, if anything, to your management of this sort of problem.

(ii) Inform the patient that he is taking his own discharge against medical advice (and, if necessary, intimate the possible risks of this action—if you can think of any). This last ditch manoeuvre may save the day.

(iii) Complete the 'Discharge Against Medical Advice' form. This is usually signed by the patient and yourself, and is witnessed by a third party (e.g. a nurse).

(iv) Record the circumstances and outcome in the patient's case notes.

In the event of a patient disregarding the above formalities and simply absconding from the ward, an appropriate member of your medical team should be contacted as a matter of urgency for such situations are stressful and require very careful handling.

4 *Discharge to accommodation other than the patient's own home* (e.g. Part III accommodation)—this arises most commonly in elderly patients and does not impinge particularly upon the houseman's workload. Most of the organization and administration is performed by the nursing staff and Social Work Department.

5 *Discharge of a patient to his home*—the uncomplicated discharge of a patient to his own home is by far the most commonly encountered situation. The following points require consideration:

(i) As always, during housejobs, foresight is essential. Anticipating a patient's discharge enables you to do much of the necessary work in advance and therefore ultimately save time. The decision to send a patient home usually evolves over the course of a few days and, thus, predicting the actual date and co-ordinating your actions appropriately are, in fact, fairly easy. Surprise discharges occur most frequently during the consultant's ward round, when your chief dismembers your treatment plan and declares that the patient may leave, 'as soon as someone can come and get him'.

(ii) An area of this subject which is grossly neglected by most housemen involves advice given to the patient when he leaves hospital. This is because junior doctors, their minds in chaos as they cram too much work into a day, tend to provide information only when it is solicited. Sadly, the patient is likely to think of possible problems which might arise on discharge (and therefore formulate appropriate questions) just as he is leaving the ward. As the houseman is rarely there 'on the spot' to wave goodbye and receive the inevitable box of chocolates, the nursing staff are left to give advice and reassurance which they would rather was proferred by the junior doctor. The message is, then, to regard instruction to the patient as mandatory and include it routinely in the list of 'essentials' when discharging a patient from hospital. Usually, all that is required is a mention of 'do's and don'ts', 'what to look out for', 'what is to be expected and ignored' and some idea of the time-scale before recovery is likely to be complete. Obviously, emphasis and detail will vary according to the particular patient (e.g. someone returning home after a myocardial infarction will require more counselling on discharge than a patient who has had an appendicectomy—although the latter will still have his fair share of anxieties which will require attention).

(iii) A patient discharged from hospital is given a 1 or 2 week supply of the drugs which he has been taking as an inpatient and which are still considered necessary for his well-being at home. Detailed instruction about the frequency and duration of treatment should be provided—especially since, in hospital, the patient has relied on the nursing staff to administer his medication. (For more information, see Chapter 8.)

(iv) You are expected to write a brief preliminary letter to the patient's GP. This entails completing a form produced specifically for this purpose and which precedes the more detailed discharge summary produced at a later date (nominally the task of your superior but frequently devolving to yourself). The patient delivers this letter to his GP as soon as possible. The information contained therein includes dates of admission and discharge; diagnosis and brief clinical details; treatment and response; drugs on discharge, with details of any modifications which might be required at a later date; plans for follow-up. In certain cases (e.g. in those who may find the transition from hospital to home a particularly major upheaval, for whatever reason) a telephone-call to the GP, in addition to the standard letter, is prudent.

(v) The follow-up arrangements (e.g. a date for an outpatient's appointment) must be made clear to the patient.

(vi) Any extra services required by the patient should be organized in advance (e.g. home-help). This is generally the province of the nursing staff and Social Services Department, but you ought to be aware, or even the instigator, of the social support intended for your patient on discharge.

22
Talking to Patients who take 'Overdoses'

The following article intentionally makes no reference to the 'medical' management of deliberate self-harm: details of that aspect of care will have to be sought elsewhere. At risk of appearing somewhat pedantic, it is probably important to state initially that there is no such thing as an 'overdose patient'; such a label fails to draw attention to the pharmacological agent involved, and contributes nothing to an understanding as to why the person in question attempted to take his life, however half-hearted that attempt may have been.

The incidence of cases of deliberate self-harm (of which approximately 90% are due to self-poisoning) has increased to such an extent that it now accounts for around 20% of general medical admissions, and probably the majority in young patients. In more easily understood, and relevant, terms this amounts to two cases per 'take' in the average district general hospital. This is obviously of some importance to yourself.

It is sad, but unfortunately true to say that 'overdose patients' often receive poor treatment in hospital, probably due to the somewhat negative attitudes of senior members of the medical profession.

Though it was officially recommended that psychological assessment should be performed by a psychiatrist, the increasing number of cases led to great strain being imposed on limited psychiatric services, and DHSS guidelines now suggest that automatic referral to a psychiatrist is no longer mandatory. What this means to you is that, faced on the one hand by the non-availability of a psychiatrist for referral, and on the other by pressure to release a bed from more senior members of your firm, you will often be left unsupervized in the evaluation of 'risk' in these individuals.

Assessment should be performed in surroundings conducive to frank discussion of personal problems; the open ward, or Casualty

Department, is not the best place: instead it should preferably be attempted in the Doctors' or Sister's offices. The interview should be attempted when the patient is medically fit; conversely though, the assessment should not be delayed unnecessarily as the patient may then have developed an unrealistic 'rationalization' of his problems, in an attempt to appear more socially acceptable.

A good plan for evaluation of patients who have engaged in deliberate self-harm is as follows:

1 Establish a rapport with the patient. Explanation of your role in assessment, together with an indication of your willingness to help, is probably all that is required in the majority of cases.

2 Attempt to understand the nature of the act, by enquiring about events in the preceding two days—factors such as the degree of planning, aims at isolation and presence of a suicide note, should be tactfully explored.

3 Difficulties perceived by the patient should be clarified—for example, problems in relationships with partners and difficulties at school or at work. An alcohol history is mandatory; there is a high level of correlation between deliberate self-harm and alcohol-related problems. Such difficulties should be placed in context by exploring the relevant personal and family background.

4 Brief psychiatric history and mental state examination should be performed in all cases—you are not expected to perform a detailed examination, but failure to ask about relevant symptoms (such as anorexia, weight loss, insomnia, feelings of hopelessness or desperation, suicidal ideation and feelings of guilt) could rightly be considered negligent.

5 Attempt to formulate with the patient a list of current problems—this enables the patient to actively participate in his subsequent management.

Plans for the future should be discussed. Elicit what the patient wants: treatment, if necessary, will be decided later.

6 Certain patients should then be referred to the psychiatric services.

It is worth mentioning here that very young patients are often unable to give a good account of themselves to an intimidating figure

Patients who take Overdoses

in a bloodstained white coat and initial assessment should then be performed by a senior member of the nursing staff, who generally are only too pleased to help with such patients.

Definitive treatment, obviously, will be decided by the psychiatrist. Though psychiatric symptoms are common in patients who have attempted to take their lives, formal psychiatric disorders are rare. This is a fact that often inspires disbelief, nevertheless experience will reveal it to be true. Far more common, however, are reports of undesirable 'life-events' such as the loss of a partner, or of employment. A patient with demonstrable mental illness and suicidal ideation would probably be admitted as a psychiatric in-patient; the majority of patients, however, will either be reviewed on an out-patient basis, or be returned to the care of the GP.

Though the above may appear, upon first reading, excessively detailed, it should prove indispensable when you find yourself somewhat confused, simultaneously acting as an entire medical team, psychiatrist, social worker, marriage guidance counsellor and provider of shoulders to cry on.

23
Ward Rounds

Ward rounds tend to be regarded with some trepidation by housemen. In fact, most rounds are brief, business-like, and demand nothing more than an ability to locate patients and scribble down instructions. Such whistle-stop tours, or 'working rounds', as they are called, are conducted by your registrar and usually occur early in the morning before the real 'working day' has begun. This article deals primarily with the more stressful 'Consultant's Round', an event which generally takes place once or twice a week.

The Consultant's round is traditionally envisaged as a rather grand and forbidding affair, especially for the junior doctors involved. Undoubtedly, this rather majestic aura evolves from a combination of factors: the houseman's memory of traumas experienced as a medical student on ward-rounds, the (in some cases) infrequent appearance of the Consultant on the ward, his possibly pyrotechnic temperament, and the inevitable respectful entourage which accompanies the round and which usually includes registrars, SHOs, senior nurses or sisters, housemen, students and peripheral staff such as physiotherapists, social workers or dieticians. Given that these ingredients confer a rather momentous and intimidating nature upon the Consultant's round, it is, perhaps, understandable that it causes housemen a good deal of anxiety.

The reality is often very different. Indeed, your task may be merely to prompt your Registrar when he cannot recall the name of a patient, and to guide the procession to the wards on which your patients reside, the rest of the time remaining a mute, attentive onlooker. Alternatively, you may be expected to 'lead' the round, presenting each patient in turn and acting as 'man on the spot' when any information is required. Clearly, it is wise to ascertain your precise role, which will probably fall somewhere between these two extremes, by

Ward Rounds

liaising with the other members of your firm prior to your ward round debut.

No matter how insignificant a part you play in the proceedings, it is vital that you have a bare minimum of information immediately to hand without having to resort to a frantic search through the patient's case notes each time you are asked a question. Such information should, therefore, be set out on a single sheet of paper which you have readily available throughout the ward round. The following plan for a very basic 'crib-sheet' is derived from those questions most commonly fired at housemen on the Consultant's tour of the ward:

For all patients
  name
  age
  occupation

For surgical patients
  diagnosis
  days pre- or post-operation
  medication
  previous operations
  any particular problems e.g. diabetes
  post-operative haemoglobin (if appropriate)
  date for discharge

For medical patients
  diagnosis
  date of admission
  past and present medication
  results of investigations performed so far
  proposed further investigations (with dates)
  treatment plan
  any particular problems
  social background (particular in the elderly)

Thus, with these facts at hand, you should remain unruffled if you are unexpectedly given the dubious honour of leading the ward round.

Simultaneously, this data sheet may be used to record the wishes of your boss with regard to suggested investigations, therapeutic regimes or other actions. These instructions are best appended in red (or in some other suitable colour) so that they may subsequently be easily extricated from the mass of information you had prepared before the ward round.

Finally a few 'Do's' and Don'ts':

Do

- Be on time for the round.
- Make sure that all patients, X-rays etc., are in their correct place prior to the round and allow none to wander from the ward (the nursing staff and ward clerk will help here).
- Ensure that the results of all vital investigations are filed in the case-notes.
- Listen to what the Consultant is saying: information imparted in a leisurely, expansive or anecdotal way to the entire audience may suddenly condense into specific instructions directed towards you.
- Sit patiently and politely drinking coffee and eating biscuits with the rest of the entourage at the end of the round, even if you have countless tasks which urgently require your attention. This is all part of ward round etiquette.

Don't

- Debate points of diagnosis or management with your boss at the patient's bedside. Even if you are correct, manners dictate that such matters are best discussed over coffee after the round. Besides, conflicting theories expounded within hearing range of the patient will do little to instil in him confidence in either Consultant or junior staff.
- Disappear to answer your bleep. This duty may be delegated to a junior nurse or medical student. Your momentary absence from the ward round often results in you failing to be informed of important

decisions regarding patient management, quite apart from any irritation it might cause your Consultant.

- Chatter excessively to the students or nurses, particularly while your consultant is talking or listening to the patient. It is astonishing how very senior ears can tune more readily to whispered details of your social life rather than a suspected gallop rhythm while auscultating a patient's heart.

- Lie to cover up your mistakes or omissions. Honesty, although sometimes excruciatingly embarrassing, is definitely the safest policy.

The Compleat Houseman

24
The Compleat Houseman

Undergraduate medical education, with its past concentration upon theoretical groundwork, almost to the exclusion of practical advice, used to render the transition from medical student to pre-registration house officer somewhat uncomfortable. This non-sequitur, from marble halls of academia to stark reality of ward practice, has to a certain extent become less disjointed with the provision of Final Year 'shadow' house officer posts and encouragement of locum appointments for students.

Unfortunately, although ward teaching appears to be occurring at ever-earlier stages of the undergraduate curriculum, exposure to consultants is likely to be restricted to formal settings, such as teaching ward rounds and outpatient clinics, which have little to do with ward management of patients—the house officer's main concern. This restriction allows you little opportunity to evaluate the interplay of roles within the medical or surgical team, and as such, you are likely to be ill-prepared to work effectively within these units, and to have little understanding of consultants' attitudes and preferences.

This section aims to clarify, admittedly to a limited extent, the requirements of consultants, by examination of the replies to a questionnaire which attempted to gauge the attitude of those who provide house jobs, in order that those yet to endure them may be marginally more prepared. The questionnaire was presented to a number of consultants in teaching and district hospitals, physicians and surgeons, in town and country. The following is not intended as an authorative analysis (the sample is small and probably non-representative) but the results are none the less illuminating.

The questionnaire included the following items, together with requests for any comments that the consultants felt pertinent.

1 Do you remember your house officers? If so, for what reasons?

2 What constitutes a 'good' house officer?
3 How frequently do you see your house officer?
4 What is the worst, or best, thing that your house officer has done?
5 Do you expect your house officers to be involved in the management of your private patients?
6 Do you feel that house officers are adequately prepared for their job?

In reply to the first question, it is interesting to note that all consultants claim to remember their house officers, though one, presumably more honest than the rest, meekly states that 'as time passes it becomes more difficult'. Reasons for such indelible imprinting are many and varied—house officers may be remembered 'for their beauty', 'for their willingness to work as hard as myself', or, somewhat perplexingly, 'because they are human beings'. Few consultants claim that mere academic prowess is a memory-jogging factor, though one claims that the main reason he is forced to remember his house officers is that 'they expect me to provide references for them, apart from anything else'. Another recalls house officers for their ability 'to take a lot of flak, be jumped on for trivial things, and be generally torn apart!'

Similarly, perceptions of what constitutes a 'good' house officer differ enormously, from one who 'does what he is told, and can be relied upon to do it', to 'one who recognizes the greater experience of the ward sister'. Legible handwriting is viewed as a redeeming factor in the otherwise undistinguished. The presumably more philosophical consultants indicate that a good houseman is one 'who has common sense, an ability to be organized, compassion, and an ability to maintain happy relationships'; one states that 'there is fundamentally no difference in dealing with medical problems in hospital than from the management of personal relationships and domestic organization'. Finally, one consultant has only limited requirements, feeling that a good house officer is one who is:

'intelligent, compassionate, courteous, industrious, obsessional, meticulous, neat, articulate, punctual, capable of forming good relationships, healthy, stable, indefatigable, ambitious . . .'

Presumably this consultant has these qualities in abundance.

The majority of consultants claim to see their house officers four or five times a week, though the period of such contact is generally unspecified. One consultant complains that he sees the house officer 'much less frequently than I would like—he spends too much time clerking admissions: I hope this will change'. It would have been interesting to compare the replies to this question from consultants to those from their respective house officers: unfortunately, the replies from the latter group were so rare as to preclude interpretation.

The worst thing a house officer can do, according to one consultant, is 'to kill my patient': the best, 'to save my patient'. Other consultants tend to view reprehensible and commendable acts less extremely, and expound with less economy of words. For example, one suggests that 'an error of judgement should always be sympathetically understood, but an error due to idleness is more culpable': another, 'consultants should be concerned with everyday qualities and not expect miracles or catastrophes' from their house officer. Reasonably, it is felt by one general surgeon that 'a smooth-running and efficient firm will not allow an inadequate house officer to make decisions that he is not capable of so doing'. There appears to be a pronounced consensus that the worst thing a house officer can do is 'to insist tests have been done, that haven't'. You have been warned. The best thing a house officer can do, according to one consultant, 'is to cheer me up at times of gloom'!

Regarding the role of the house officer in the management of private patients, the majority of those consultants who have a private practice feel that there should be some involvement from the house officer. Those consultants working in academic departments require that this be so, as the revenue funds research. One orthopaedic surgeon regards experience of private medicine as 'an essential part of training', another surgeon states, humbly, that 'private patients get better treatment if the house officer is involved'. There is a general agreement, however, that the private sector should *not* be a prime feature of the job or training.

It is interesting to note that the replies to the final question 'do you feel that house officers are adequately prepared for their job?' is the source of greatest controversy, and that there is an exact fifty-fifty split between those who feel housemen are prepared, and those who do not. One surgeon glibly states that 'house officers are not prepared—and never have been'; many feel that the post is a training post and that considerations of preparation are of only peripheral importance. A physician states that house officers would be marginally more prepared for the onslaught if 'their heads were less overstuffed with academic rubbish'; another that house officers are 'ill-prepared to cope with the organization'. Finally, one teaching hospital head of department states that 'I don't think *any* curriculum within *any* medical school can prepare *any* human being for the task'.

The role of the house officer as 'final common pathway' and main organ of communication in the ward management of patients has been stressed frequently in this book. It is probably unremarkable, then, that this aspect of the house officer's job is considered by nursing staff to be the most important. In an attempt to understand what nurses regard as essential qualities in the house officer, a questionnaire was presented to a number of nurses, of various grades, working in a variety of hospitals. The following areas of enquiry were included.
1 On the whole, do you find housemen sympathetic to the nursing staff?
2 What to you feel are good qualities in a house officer?
3 What are the faults of a bad houseman?
4 Do patients get a good deal from house officers?
5 Do housemen get a good deal from the senior members of the medical team?
6 Do house officers ever jeopardize the well-being of patients? If so, how?

Again, the results from this questionnaire were probably too limited to allow definitive 'analysis', but general inferences may be drawn. It appears that the majority of nurses feel that house officers *are* sensitive and sympathetic to the needs of the nursing staff, and that houseladies rather than housemen are more likely to be perceptive of the nurses' requirements.

'Good' qualities in a houseman include general features such as effective communication, patience, flexibility and punctiliousness, together with rather more specific attributes such as ability to conform to age-decreed ward routine, efficiency in the institution of intravenous access, and willingness to see relatives. 'Good' housemen, it is said, answer their bleeps promptly.

Conversely, house officers likely to be regarded, by nurses, as 'bad' are those who fail to answer their bleeps readily: one wonders how junior doctors were judged prior to the development of this particular gadget. Undesirable qualities in the house officer also include absconding from the ward after practical procedures, without offering to help clear up detritus; failure to anticipate, and prepare for a patient's discharge; and inability to smile when it is considered generally appropriate so to do.

Patients get a 'good deal' from house officers in the opinion of the nursing staff. Regrettably, however, the majority of nurses feel that, while adequate guidance and support may generally be provided by the registrar, the consultants' expectations of house officers tend to be rather unrealistic.

House officers have, fortunately, been seen to jeopardize patient well-being only very occasionally, and the nursing staff appear to have much sympathy, citing long working hours and inadequate supervision as contributory factors to mismanagement. Failure to respond to anguished pleas from experienced ward nurses, only too well aware of deterioration in a patient's clinical condition is—rightly—considered culpable, and repeated attempts by the inexperienced house officer at difficult practical procedures is viewed adversely.

It is probably impossible to perpetually satisfy all interested parties, each with particular expectations of, and idiosyncratic attitudes towards, house officers: good communication skills, and heightened powers of perception, however, probably render such a herculean task somewhat more achievable—as should this guidebook.

Clerking

25
History and Examination Framework

The following exists as both an *aide-mémoire* to rapid but thorough clerking and a survey of medical record hieroglyphics. Although the latter are probably vaguely familiar to all but the most naive of fledgling housemen, remarkable variation in symbolism does occur. In addition, a basic guide of this sort is undoubtedly of great interest to medical students who are all too often confronted with the condensed and abbreviated notes of a busy superior which they then have to decipher. Everyone has their own favourite shorthand, and although much is universally 'accepted', vital pieces of information can sometimes be concealed behind someone's pet abbreviation.

History

1 Name
2 Age
3 Occupation
4 Marital status
5 Route of referral e.g. emergency, via clinic, routine, etc.
6 Presenting complaint (C/O = 'complains of')—in brief, and, preferably, in the patient's own words.
7 History of presenting complaint (HPC)
8 Past medical history (PH), which usually comprises:
- any similar previous episodes of this presenting complaint
- past operations
- past illnesses
- current and past medication
- known drug allergies or idiosyncrasies

9 Family history (FH) e.g.
- hereditary diseases

- familial tendency to disease, with special reference towards the patient's presenting complaint
- concurrent (and possibly similar) illness in the family; this is relevant, for example, in suspected infectious disease

10 Social history (SH)
  - home background
  - social service provision
  - smoking habits
  - drinking habits

11 Systems' review (SR, or DQ = 'direct questioning')—a brief and fairly comprehensive interrogation, such as described below:

Cardiovascular system (CVS)
- shortness of breath on exercise (SOBOE)?
- orthopnoea?
- paroxysmal nocturnal dyspnoea (PND)?
- angina?
- palpitations?
- swelling of ankles (SOA)?
- claudication?

Respiratory system (RS)
- shortness of breath?
- wheezing?
- cough?
- sputum/haemoptysis?

Gastrointestinal tract (GIT)
- weight changes?
- appetite changes?
- abdominal pain?
- nausea or vomiting?
- change in bowel habit?
- rectal bleeding?

Urogenital system (UG):
Males ● prostatic symptoms, such as hesitancy, poor stream and post-micturition dribbling (PMD)?
Females ● menstrual history

History and Examination

- abnormal vaginal bleeding or discharge?

Males and Females • dysuria or haematuria?

Central nervous system (CNS)
- headaches?
- weakness?
- fits?
- faints?
- paraesthesiae?

Notes

1 The overall emphasis of a history should be tailored towards the presenting complaint. Questions are designed to elicit information which will contribute towards formulation of a rational diagnosis and its probable aetiology. For example, in a case of suspected chronic liver disease, you might (in addition to other appropriate enquiries) question the patient rather more closely than usual about alcohol intake. In the same case, occupation (e.g. publican, company executive, doctor, etc.) might be particularly relevant.

This shifting of emphasis should be employed in other situations. It is obviously far more important to know, in detail, the home situation—under 'social history'—of an elderly patient with crippling arthritis (e.g. type of housing, stairs, presence of other people at home, support from relatives, friends, neighbours and social services) than it is in the case of a young, fit man attending routinely for removal of an ingrowing toenail.

Thus, the 'History Framework' should be regarded as a flexible tool designed to highlight the pertinent points of a patient's medical, psychological and social background.

2 In the 'Past Medical History' section, apart from enquiry into previous operations and a general question regarding any serious illnesses, certain medical conditions are, usually, specifically sought. These often include:
- ischaemic heart disease
- hypertension

- tuberculosis
- diabetes mellitus
- rheumatic fever
- epilepsy

In medical shorthand, presuming each enquiry is negative, this is transformed into

°IHD °HT (or ° ↑ BP) °TB °DM °RhF °Ep

3 All too often, a patient is labelled as, 'allergic to drug X', when, in fact, drug X simply once made him feel sick or gave him diarrhoea. Such reactions are better noted as idiosyncrasies or intolerances. True allergies should be highlighted in the notes and recorded on the front of the patient's drug sheet and, ideally, on the cover of the patient's case notes.

4 Abbreviations and jargon afflict history recording only mildly (especially when compared to 'On Examination' notes). The 'System Review' section may be the most difficult to decode as much of it is written in medical shorthand.

5 Usually, as in the framework above, symptoms of musculoskeletal, endocrine, dermatological or psychiatric problems are not solicited unless:

(i) The patient's illness could feasibly be linked with one of these systems

(ii) You are performing a particularly detailed medical history.

Similarly, gynaecological questioning is often minimal unless it would appear appropriate to be more thorough.

6 It has been suggested that the following brief and vague questions are quite sufficient to ensure that no major pathology is overlooked in the 'Systems Review', particularly in a rapid 'surgical' clerking:

(i) Have you had any loss of appetite?
(ii) Have you had any loss of weight?
(iii) Do you suffer from chest pain?
(iv) Do you suffer from shortness of breath?
(v) Are your 'waterworks' functioning normally?
(vi) Are your bowels functioning normally?

Examination

Examination of a 'specimen patient'—a healthy, cooperative young woman. NB Such a patient rarely exists.

Notation	**Explanation**
O/E	*On Examination*
Fit-looking, cooperative young woman.	Brief description of patient.
°JAClCyL	No jaundice, anaemia, clubbing, cyanosis or lymphadenopathy.
Apyrexial	Temperature normal.
CVS	*Cardiovascular system*
Pulse 70 reg., good vol.	Pulse rate and character.
Blood pressure 120/80	Blood pressure.
JVP ⟷	Jugular venous pressure not raised.
AB 5th ICSMCL	Apex beat in fifth intercostal space, mid-clavicular line. (Alternative—AB N/D i.e. not displaced)
HS I—II +nil	Heart sounds one and two normal, with no added sounds.
°oedema	No oedema.
PPs √ °bruits	Peripheral pulses present. No bruits. (Alternative—sketch of 'matchstick man' with + for pulse present and 0 or − for pulse absent.)
Resp	*Respiratory system*
Trachea ↓	Trachea central.
Expansion good + =	Expansion good and equal each side.
Percussion res + =	Percussion resonant and equal each side.
BS vesic. + nil added.	Breath sounds vesicular; no added sounds.
VF } NAD VR	Vocal fremitus and resonance normal.

Abdo.

Soft

°masses
°scars
°tenderness
°LK$_2$S

BS √
HO's √
PR–NAD

Abdomen

Abdomen soft with no masses, scars or tenderness.

Liver, kidneys and spleen not palpable.
Bowel sounds present and normal.
Hernial orifices normal.
Rectal examination normal.

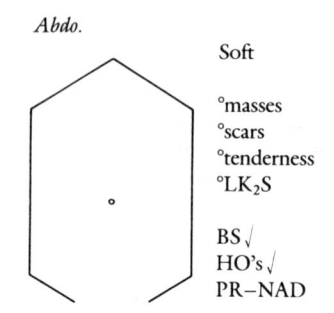

Breasts

Breasts

Breasts represented diagrammatically, each divided into quadrants, examined and recorded separately. Axillary and cervical lymph node areas similarly depicted.

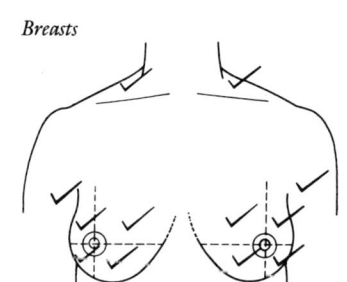

CNS
Orientated T+S

PERLA

Fundi–NAD
Cranials II–XII intact

Arms: power
  tone
  sensation
  coordination } NAD
Reflexes: B T S
  r. + + +
  l. + + +

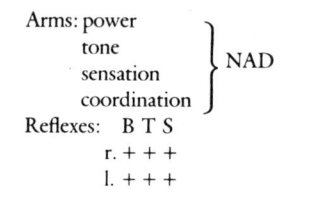

Central nervous system
Orientated in time and space.
(Alternative—orientated TPP—i.e. orientated in time, place and person.)
Pupils equal and reacting to light and accommodation.
Fundi–normal.
Second to twelfth cranial nerves normal (N.B. First cranial nerve rarely tested routinely).
Power, tone, sensation and coordination normal in upper limbs.

Biceps, triceps, and supinator reflexes present and equal in both arms.

Legs: power ⎫
     tone ⎬ NAD
     sensation ⎪
     coordination ⎭

Power, tone, sensation and coordination normal in lower limbs.

Reflexes: K A Pl
    r. + + ↓
    l. + + ↓

Knee and ankle reflexes present and equal in legs. Plantar reflexes downwards on both sides.

°clonus — No clonus.
°cerebellar signs — No cerebellar signs.

Notes

1 Orthopaedic/detailed joint examination is usually omitted unless appropriate.
2 Vaginal examination is usually omitted except when it might provide useful information, for example in a woman with lower abdominal pain.
3 Surgical clerkings, especially when performed in a hurry, can become fairly minimal such that the CNS is reported as 'grossly normal' (implying that the patient can talk and walk—although, in fact, the latter is rarely formally tested!). Similarly, although the other systems are examined thoroughly, they are recorded, if normal, rather briefly, for example—
CVS—unremarkable (with pulse and BP readings)
Resp—clear
Abdo—NAD
4 The emphasis of the physical examination is tailored towards the presenting complaint.

Common variations from the normal

This section describes the medical symbols and shorthands used to depict the most common variations from the norm.

Jaundiced — Often recorded as icteric.
Lymphadenopathy — Either written description of enlarged lymph-nodes, or 'matchstick-man' body to depict areas of lymphadenopathy.
CNs—cervical nodes
ANs—axillary nodes
SCNs—supraclavicular nodes
INs—inguinal nodes

Chapter 25

CVS
JVP ↑ 4 cm

AB N/P
AAL/MAL/PAL

HS I—∿∿∿—II
   ↑
   ESM → neck
   loudest AA
HS I∿∿∿∿II
   ↑
   PSM → axilla

Peripheral pulses

Cardiovascular system
Jugular venous pressure raised 4 cm from the sternal angle.
Apex beat not palpable
In anterior axillary line, mid-axillary line, posterior axillary line.
Heart sounds with ejection systolic murmur, radiating to neck, heard loudest in aortic area.

Heart sounds with pansystolic murmur radiating to axilla.

NB. Murmur loudness is often 'graded' out of six, e.g. 3/6—moderately loud.
Often recorded diagrammatically as already described. Bruits sometimes depicted thus:

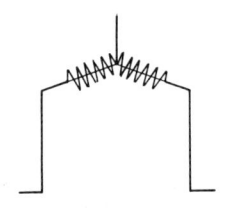

Resp.
Trachea → r.
         l. ←
Expansion   ⎫
Percussion   ⎬ ↓ l.
Breath sounds ⎪
Creps   ⎭

Rhonchi

Respiratory system
Trachea deviated to right/left.

Poor expansion, dull percussion and decreased breath sounds on the left.

Crepitations (crackling, interrupted sounds)
Wheezes.

History and Examination

Abdo.

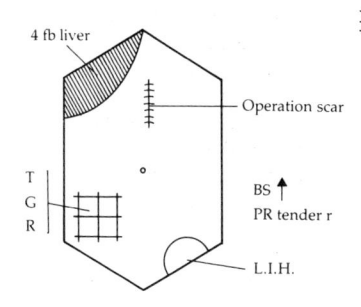

Abdomen

▦ to localize area of abnormality

Liver enlarged to four finger breadths below the costal margin (although should really be measured in cm).

Rectal examination tender on right side.

Left inguinal hernia.

TGR—tenderness, guarding and rebound—often crudely graded as +, ++ or +++.

BS ↑—increased bowel sounds.

Breasts

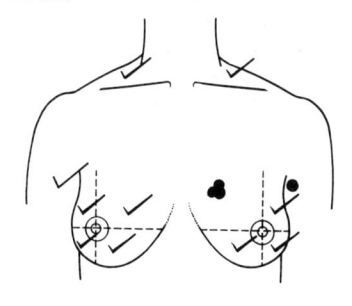

♣ represents breast lump
● represents lymph node, both of which are described in the usual way, viz. size, shape, consistency, fixation, etc.

CNS

Pl ↑ ↑—bilateral upgoing plantars (Babinski's sign).

Abnormalities are usually described in full, for example, hyperreflexia left side (often coarsely graded as absent, +, ++, +++), reduced power on right (sometimes recorded quantitatively using a 0–5 grading system), etc.

26
Abbreviations

Any attempted 'dictionary' of medical shorthand cannot hope to be comprehensive, for the written format of medical notation evolves naturally with time and the individual's idiosyncrasies. The following exists, therefore, not to encourage abbreviation and symbolism, but, hopefully, to guide those (namely housemen and medical students) most commonly perplexed by it.

Much of medical shorthand is specific to areas of history and examination recording. These abbreviations (such as 'HS' for 'heart sounds' and 'PN' for 'percussion note', etc.) appear consistently in the detailing of a full clerking, and, as such, are explained in the 'History and Examination Framework' section. For this reason, they will not be repeated here.

Medical specialities such as Obstetrics and Gynaecology, Paediatrics and Psychiatry have their own batch of hieroglyphics. These are omitted because such specialities generally involve the post-registration doctor.

Essentially, the list produced below is simply representative of those abbreviations which we have encountered most often or found most baffling.

Medical Abbreviations and Symbols

AA	Australia antigen
AAA	abdominal aortic aneurysm
ABGs	arterial blood gases
AF	atrial fibrillation
AFB	acid-fast bacilli (as in tuberculosis)
ANF	anti-nuclear factor
AP	anteroposterior

Abbreviations

ARF	acute renal failure
ASD	atrial septal defect
AXR (e&s)	abdominal X-ray (erect and supine)
Ba	barium (as in barium meal, etc.)
BBB	bundle branch block
BCC	basal cell carcinoma
BD	twice a day
BID	brought in dead
BM	bone marrow
BNF	British National Formulary
BO (R)	bowels open (regularly)
BP	blood pressure
BPH	benign prostatic hypertrophy
Bx	biopsy
CA or Ca	carcinoma
CABG	coronary artery bypass graft
CAT	computerized axial tomography (as 'CAT scan', often shortened to 'CT' scan)
CCF	congestive cardiac failure
CCU	coronary care unit
CDs	controlled drugs (= DDAs)
CGL	chronic granulocytic leukaemia
C_2H_5OH	alcohol
CLL	chronic lymphocytic leukaemia
COAD	chronic obstructive airways disease
CRF	chronic renal failure
CSF	cerebro-spinal fluid
CSU	catheter specimen of urine
CVA	cerebro-vascular accident
CXR	chest X-ray
D & V	diarrhoea and vomiting
DDAs	dangerous drugs act (refers to controlled drugs = CDs)

DIPJ	distal interphalangeal joint
DLE	discoid lupus erythematosus
DM	diabetes mellitus
DNA	did not attend
DOA	dead on arrival
DU	duodenal ulcer
DVT	deep vein thrombosis
D/W	discussed with
DXT	deep X-ray therapy
ECG	electrocardiogram
ECT	electro convulsive therapy
EEG	electroencephalogram
EMG	electromyogram
EMU	early morning urine
ERCP	endoscopic retrograde cholangio-pancreatogram
ESR	erythrocyte sedimentation rate
FBC	full blood count
FEV_1	forced expiratory volume in one second
FOBs	faecal occult bloods
FROM	full range of movement
FTA	fluorescent treponemal antibody (syphilis serology)
FVC	forced vital capacity
GA	general anaesthetic
G&S	group and save
GI (T)	gastrointestinal (tract)
GTN	glyceryl trinitrate
GU	gastric ulcer
HH	hiatus hernia
HI	head injury

HIV	human immunodeficiency virus
HL	Hodgkin's lymphoma
HT	hypertension (sometimes as ↑ BP)
Hx	haemorrhage
ICU	intensive care unit (= ITU)
IDD	insulin dependent diabetic
IH	inguinal hernia
IHD	ischaemic heart disease
IM	intramuscular
ISQ	no change (in status quo)
ITU	intensive therapy unit (= ICU)
IV	intravenous
IVI	intravenous infusion
IVP	intravenous pyelogram (= IVU)
IVU	intravenous urogram (= IVP)
Ix	investigations
KOd	knocked out
LA	local anaesthetic
LFTs	liver function tests
LMN	lower motor neurones
LMP	last menstrual period
LN	lymph node
LP	lumbar puncture
Mané	in the morning
MAOIs	monoamine oxidase inhibitors
MI	myocardial infarction
Mims	drugs booklet
Mitotic lesion	cancer
MS	multiple sclerosis
MS (S) U	mid-stream (specimen of) urine
MCPJ	metacarpophalangeal joint

NAD	no abnormality detected (or, to the cynics, 'not actually done')
NAI	non-accidental injury
NBI	no bony injury
NBM	nil by mouth
Neisserial infection	gonorrhoea
NFR	not for resuscitation
NG	new growth, i.e. cancer
NHL	non-Hodgkin's lymphoma
NIDD	non insulin dependent diabetic
nocté	at night
NSAID	non steroidal anti-inflammatory drug
NSR	no sign of recurrence
OA	osteoarthritis
OD	once a day
OD	overdose
OGD	oesophagogastroduodenoscopy
OPA	outpatients appointment
Open and shut	inoperable case
PA	posteroanterior
PE	pulmonary embolism
PEFR	peak expiratory flow rate
PID	pelvic inflammatory disease
PID	prolapsed intervertebral disc
PIPJ	proximal interphalangeal joint
PM	post mortem
PMD	post micturition dribbling
PND	paroxysmal nocturnal dyspnoea
PO	per oram (drug route)
PP	private patient
PR	per rectum
PRN	as required
PTC	percutaneous transhepatic cholangiogram

PUO	pyrexia of unknown origin
PV	per vagina
PVD	peripheral vascular disease
Px	prescription or prescribe
QDS	four times a day
RA	rheumatoid arthritis
RBS (G)	random blood sugar (glucose)
Rh F	rheumatic fever
ROM	range of movement
RT	radiotherapy
RTA	road traffic accident
RTI	respiratory tract infection
Rx	treatment or treat
S/B	seen by
SBE	subacute bacterial endocarditis
SC	subcutaneous
SCC	squamous cell carcinoma
SL	sublingual
SLE	systemic lupus erythematosus
SOA	swelling of ankles
SOB (OE)	shortness of breath (on exercise)
SOL	space occupying lesion
SR	sinus rhythm
STD	sexually transmitted disease
Supratentorial	'in the mind'
SVC	superior vena cava (as in 'SVC obstruction')
SVT	supraventricular tachycardia
SXR	skull X-ray
TCAD	tricyclic antidepressant
TCI	to come in
TKVO	to keep vein open

TDS	three times a day
TEDs	thromboembolic deterrents (type of stocking)
TFTs	thyroid function tests
THR	total hip replacement
TIA	transient ischaemic attack
tissued	describes an intravenous line in which fluid is leaking into the tissues surrounding a vein
TLC	'tender loving care' i.e. analgesia and careful inactivity in terminal care
TLE	temporal lobe epilepsy
T/N/M	tumour/nodes/metastases (tumour grading system)
TPHA	treponema pallidum haemagglutination (syphilis serology)
TPN	total parenteral nutrition
T/P/R	temperature/pulse/respiration (nursing observations)
Treponemal infection	syphilis
Ts & As	tonsils and adenoids
TTAs	'to take aways' (refers to discharge drugs = TTOs)
TTOs	'to take outs' (= TTAs)
U & Es	urea and electrolytes
UMN	upper motor neurone
URTI	respiratory tract infection
U/S	ultrasound
UT	urinary tract
UTI	urinary tract infection
VDRL	venereal disease research laboratory (syphilis serology)
VF	ventricular fibrillation
VMI	very much improved

Abbreviations

VQ	ventilation-perfusion (as in VQ scan)
VSD	ventricular septal defect
VT	ventricular tachycardia
VVs	varicose veins
WR	ward round
WR	Wassermann reaction (syphilis serology)
X-match	cross-match
XR	X-ray
$\because$	because
$\triangle$	diagnosis
†	died
$\triangle\triangle$	differential diagnosis
#	fracture
-ve	negative
°	no (as in °SOB = no shortness of breath)
$\longleftrightarrow$	no change (as in weight, 'weight steady')
+ve	positive
1°	primary (2°—secondary etc.)
Σ	sigmoidoscopy
†, †† etc.	one tablet, two tablets, etc.
$\therefore$	therefore
$\odot$	unit
$\bar{c}$	with
1/7	one day
2/52	two weeks
3/12	three months

Index

Abbreviations 142–9
Abdominal surgery 19
Administrator 75, 78
AIDS 20
Alcohol 10, 26, 51, 72, 84, 116
Allergies 10, 57, 136
Anaesthetist 13, 31, 93
'Antibiotic cover' 19, 20
Arterial puncture 94–5

Bleep 64–5, 109, 120–1, 129
Blood gases 94–5
Blood transfusion 44–6
Brie 63

Cannulae 41–2, 60, 68, 91–3
Casualty 23, 66–7
Catheters, urinary 93–4
Chronic obstructive airways disease 19
Clerking 9–11, 25–7, 133–41
Compleat Houseman, the 125–9
Confidentiality 77–8
Confusion 50–2, 111
Consent 13, 56, 67, 75–7
Coroner 55, 56
Cottage hospital 35
'Crash calls' 30–3, 53
Cremation form 56
Cross-matching 12
Cystoscopy 20

Death 53–6, 99
Death certificate 55–6
'Death warmed up' 70, 73

Defibrillator 32
Diabetic patients 18–19, 58
Discharge drugs 60, 113
Discharge from hospital 107–8, 112–14, 129
Discharge letter 113–14
Discharge summary 7, 113
Drug charts 57–60, 67, 97
Drug lunch 62–3
Drug reps. 61–3, 72
Dying patient 27, 29, 33, 47–9, 86–7

ECG 7, 12, 82, 97
Elective surgery 8–22
Endotracheal tube 31, 32
Excuses and ruses 64–70

Femoral stab 93

'Group and save' 7, 45, 93

Heparinization 20
History-taking 133–6

Idiosyncracies, Consultant 15, 70
Insomnia 71–4
Intensive Care Unit 21
Intravenous drugs 81, 96–7
Intravenous infusions 16, 17, 42–4, 57–8
Investigations 11, 17, 27–9, 68–9, 104

Index

Jaundice 20

Kardex 33, 81

Legalities 75–79

Medical Defence Body 75, 79
Medical patient, the 25–37
Medical student 64, 69

Nasogastric feeding 85
Nasogastric tubes 19, 95–6
Negligence 78–9
Night sedation 52, 57, 59, 72
'Not for resuscitation' 33–4
Nursing hierarchy 80–2
Nursing officer 53, 82
Nutrition 58, 83–7

Observations, nursing 8, 46, 80
'On-call' rota 4
'On take' 23–4, 66–7
Operative care 16
'Outliers' 66
Overdoses 115–17

Past medical history 133, 135–6
Patients' Affairs Officer 55, 56
Peripheral staff 88–90
Post-mortem 56
Post-operative care 16–17
Post-operative complications 17
Post-operative investigations 17
Post-operative medication 14, 17, 59
Practical dilemmas 91–6
'Pre-med.' 13, 14, 57
Pre-operative investigations 11–12, 18–20
Preparation for housejobs 3–6, 127–8
Priorities 99
Private patients 55, 100–2, 127
'Problem-orientated' approach 36–7

Referals 103–5
Relatives 48, 55, 106–9
'Resource book' 35
Routes of exit 110–14

Self-discharge 111–12
'Social admissions' 34–6, 68
Social history 134, 135
Surgical patient, the 8–24
'Systems Review' 134–5, 136

'Talking heads' 84
Theatre-list 16
'Tissuing' 42, 92
Total parenteral nutrition 44, 83, 85–6
Transfers 24, 68, 110
Transfusion reaction 46

Venesection 93

'Ward book' 4
Ward diary 14
Ward round 73, 118–21